100 Questions & Answers About Kidney Dialysis

Lawrence E. Stam, MD
New York Methodist Hospital
The Rogosin Institute

JONES AND BARTLETT PUBLISHERS
Sudbury, Massachusetts
BOSTON   TORONTO   LONDON   SINGAPORE

World Headquarters

Jones and Bartlett Publishers
40 Tall Pine Drive
Sudbury, MA 01776
978-443-5000
info@jbpub.com
www.jbpub.com

Jones and Bartlett Publishers
Canada
6339 Ormindale Way
Mississauga, Ontario L5V 1J2
Canada

Jones and Bartlett Publishers
International
Barb House, Barb Mews
London W6 7PA
United Kingdom

Jones and Bartlett's books and products are available through most bookstores and online booksellers. To contact Jones and Bartlett Publishers directly, call 800-832-0034, fax 978-443-8000, or visit our website, www.jbpub.com.

Substantial discounts on bulk quantities of Jones and Bartlett's publications are available to corporations, professional associations, and other qualified organizations. For details and specific discount information, contact the special sales department at Jones and Bartlett via the above contact information or send an email to specialsales@jbpub.com.

The authors, editor, and publisher have made every effort to provide accurate information. However, they are not responsible for errors, omissions, or for any outcomes related to the use of the contents of this book and take no responsibility for the use of the products and procedures described. Treatments and side effects described in this book may not be applicable to all people; likewise, some people may require a dose or experience a side effect that is not described herein. Drugs and medical devices are discussed that may have limited availability controlled by the Food and Drug Administration (FDA) for use only in a research study or clinical trial. Research, clinical practice, and government regulations often change the accepted standard in this field. When consideration is being given to use of any drug in the clinical setting, the healthcare provider or reader is responsible for determining FDA status of the drug, reading the package insert, and reviewing prescribing information for the most up-to-date recommendations on dose, precautions, and contraindications, and determining the appropriate usage for the product. This is especially important in the case of drugs that are new or seldom used.

Production Credits
Executive Publisher: Christopher Davis
Senior Editorial Assistant: Jessica Acox
Production Director: Amy Rose
Production Editors: Rachel Rossi/Laura Almozara
Manufacturing and Inventory Supervisor: Amy Bacus
Composition: Paw Print Media
Cover Design: Carolyn Downer
Cover Images: Top left photo: © Carme Balcells/ShutterStock, Inc.; Top right photo: © Monkey Business Images/ShutterStock, Inc.; Middle photo: © Daniel Mirer/New York Methodist Hospital; Bottom photo: © iofotopub/ShutterStock, Inc.
Printing and Binding: Malloy, Inc.
Cover Printing: Malloy, Inc.

Library of Congress Cataloging-in-Publication Data
Stam, Lawrence E.
  100 questions and answers about kidney dialysis / Lawrence E. Stam.
    p. cm.
  Includes bibliographical references.
  ISBN-13: 978-0-7637-5417-4 (alk. paper)
  ISBN-10: 0-7637-5417-X
  1. Hemodialysis—Popular works. I. Title. II. Title: One hundred questions and answers about kidney dialysis.
  RC901.7.H45S67 2010
  617.4'61059—dc22
                              2008052442

6048

Printed in the United States of America
13 12 11 10 09   10 9 8 7 6 5 4 3 2 1

To my wife Claudia, the great love of my life now and always.

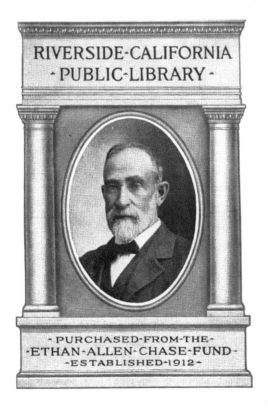

Contents

All of us know someone with kidney disease. Many of us have a friend or a family member on dialysis. This is because the number of people in the United States and the developing world with kidney disease is growing rapidly. In 2006 in the United States, 500,000 patients received some form of end-stage renal disease therapy. The Medicare cost to treat kidney disease was $23 billion.

Patients with kidney disease get a great deal of advice from well-meaning friends and family members. They are encouraged to drink more fluids to flush out the kidneys or to drink cranberry juice. Much of this advice is wrong.

The most common reaction to learning that one has kidney disease is fear. Patients are afraid of dying, of suffering pain and disability, and of the unknown impact that kidney disease and dialysis will have on their lives.

100 Questions & Answers About Kidney Dialysis is a user-friendly guide to kidney disease and dialysis. It gives basic information about kidney disease in language that is comprehensible to people without a scientific or healthcare background. It will help patients who are facing dialysis treatments learn what to expect and help prepare them for beginning dialysis treatments. The book's candid treatment of difficult questions such as "How long can I live on dialysis?" is designed to encourage patients to discuss important and difficult issues with their doctors and families. The more knowledge a patient has about kidney disease, the less fear he or she will have about starting treatment.

Dialysis was one of the most significant medical achievements of the twentieth century. Dialysis is life sustaining and improves the quality of patients' lives. It is important to remember that dialysis treatments have only been available to large numbers of patients for the past 40 years. The forces of globalization and economic development are bringing dialysis treatments to more patients and to areas of the world where dialysis has not been available before. The continued improvement in dialysis machines, dialysis membranes, new medications, and our understanding of kidney failure will result in significant improvement in dialysis treatments during the twenty-first century.

Acknowledgments

The process of writing *100 Questions & Answers About Kidney Dialysis* involved continuing conversations with several patients receiving dialysis treatments at the Rogosin Brooklyn Dialysis Unit, located at the New York Methodist Hospital in Brooklyn, New York. These conversations were invaluable in looking at kidney disease in new ways and developing creative strategies to face dialysis treatments. I would especially like to thank Erick Lucero, Henry Spellman, George Garcia, and Yoshi Reynolds for their hard work on this book. Staff members at the Rogosin Brooklyn Dialysis Unit helped provide expert information in their fields. Robin Grande, LMSW; Lisa Modica, RD, CDN; Ellen DeMarco, RN, MSN, MBA; Vera Auerbach; and Kotresha Neelakantappa, MD, all worked hard to make this book possible. Thank you Roxanna Bologa, MD, for your guidance on peritoneal dialysis. My wife Claudia S. Plottel, MD, gave me constant support, encouragement, and technical assistance.

PART ONE

The Basics

What do the kidneys do?

Where are the kidneys located?

Can kidney disease be inherited?

More ...

1. What do the kidneys do?

The **kidneys** are a pair of internal organs that are each the size of a fist. They are composed of several different types of tissues including blood vessels, tubules, and supporting structures. The purpose of the large blood vessels is to carry blood to and from the kidney. Smaller blood vessels, called capillaries, filter the blood of water, salts, toxins, and medications. Once the blood is filtered, kidney tubules can reabsorb or secrete water, salts, or other substances based upon the needs of our body. On a very hot day, we can reabsorb much of the filtered water and salt to prevent dehydration. If we overeat and drink at a holiday party, our kidneys can eliminate extra water and salt to prevent us from becoming overloaded. Fluid and salt in the urine are carried by a collecting system resembling a funnel to tubes called the ureters. The ureters carry the urine to the bladder where it can be stored until a convenient time for us to urinate.

In addition to the elimination process, there are cells in the kidney that make protein messengers called hormones. One of these hormones, **erythropoietin**, tells our bone marrow to make more red blood cells. Other cells store energy from the carbohydrates in the food we eat in the form of a polysaccharide called **glycogen**. Some kidney cells break down medications we take such as antibiotics and insulin to remove them from our bodies, which prevents us from accumulating too much medication. Many of the jobs our kidneys perform for us are unknown and are just now being discovered by scientists.

Kidneys

Two fist-sized organs located in the posterior upper abdomen that maintain fluid and salt balance and detoxify the blood by eliminating toxins and poisons from the body in the urine.

Erythropoietin

A hormone produced by the kidneys that signals the bone marrow to produce more red blood cells. In kidney disease, less erythropoietin is produced and anemia can occur. Erythropoietin can be given by injection to treat anemia.

Glycogen

A polysaccharide composed of glucose, which is the principal storage unit of carbohydrates in the body.

2. Where are the kidneys located?

Most people have two functioning kidneys. They are located in the abdomen in the lumbar region of the back, right under the lungs (**Figure 1**). They are partially protected by the rib cage. Occasionally a person can be born with one kidney or one normal kidney and another that is small and not working. Another condition, known as **horseshoe kidney**, occurs when a person is born with a single large kidney. Most of the time people with one kidney or a horseshoe kidney have no symptoms. Patients who have a horseshoe kidney or a single kidney are often discovered when **ultrasound** or **computed axial tomography (CT)** scans are done for

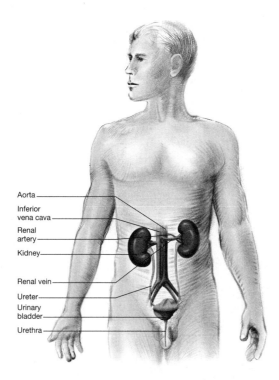

Aorta
Inferior vena cava
Renal artery
Kidney
Renal vein
Ureter
Urinary bladder
Urethra

Figure 1 Kidney location

Source: Robert K. Clark, *Anatomy and Physiology: Understanding the Human Body.* ©2005, Jones and Bartlett LLC.

The Basics

Horseshoe kidney
A medical condition in which the right and left kidneys are fused at the upper or lower pole. Ninety percent of horseshoe kidneys are fused at the lower pole. The horseshoe kidney is capable of normal kidney function and is usually found when a CT scan or ultrasound (sonogram) is performed for abdominal pain or other symptoms. Patients with a horseshoe kidney are not predisposed to kidney disease.

Ultrasound
An ultrasound, also known as a sonogram, is a diagnostic test that bounces sound waves off internal organs, such as the kidneys, to obtain a picture of them.

Computed axial tomography (CT)
A computer generated three-dimensional x-ray picture of part of the body used for the diagnosis of disease. It is sometimes called a CT scan.

other reasons. Many times when we have pain in our back, we think it is due to a kidney problem. More likely, back pain is caused by muscle strain or spasm, or a vertebral disc problem. Pain in the back that radiates to the side or into the groin can be due to a kidney stone.

3. What is the glomerulus?

Glomerulus

The part of the kidney composed of small blood vessels that filters the blood to produce urine.

The kidneys are composed of about two million functional units called nephrons. A nephron is composed of a glomerulus, kidney tubules, and blood vessels. A **glomerulus** can be thought of as a small filter. It is made up of small blood vessels called capillaries. Blood comes to the glomerulus from larger blood vessels

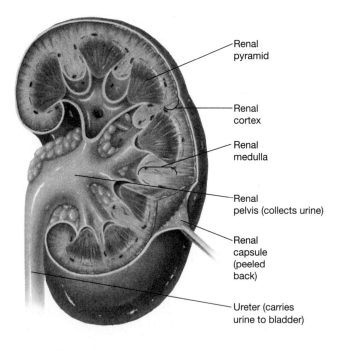

Renal pyramid

Renal cortex

Renal medulla

Renal pelvis (collects urine)

Renal capsule (peeled back)

Ureter (carries urine to bladder)

Figure 1 cont'd.

Source: Robert K. Clark, *Anatomy and Physiology: Understanding the Human Body.* ©2005, Jones and Bartlett LLC.

called the renal arteries, which then branch into smaller and smaller blood vessels until they meet the glomeruli, which are one cell thick (**Figure 2**). Fluid, salts, sugars, and small substances can pass through the thin wall of the glomerulus, but larger substances such as proteins, red blood cells, and white blood cells are too big to be filtered. If the glomerulus is damaged, proteins or blood cells can find their way through the glomerulus and into the urine. This problem can be discovered by having a test called a urine analysis, which can be done at any medical laboratory. Often the first sign of kidney problems is discovered because a routine urine analysis done for a yearly physical, an application for life insurance, or for an employment physical contains protein or blood.

We can live a normal life with a reduced number of glomeruli. People who have a kidney removed surgi-

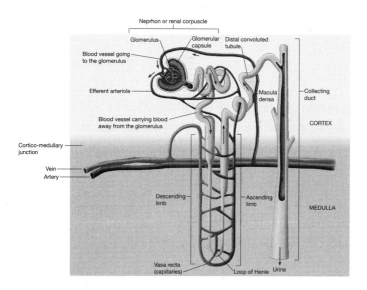

Figure 2 The functioning units of the kidney

Source: Robert K. Clark, *Anatomy and Physiology: Understanding the Human Body.* ©2005, Jones and Bartlett LLC.

Hypertrophy

An increase in the size of the kidney.

Diabetes

A disease characterized by an elevation of the glucose level in the blood. This can be caused by a decrease in insulin production by the pancreas or a defect in the insulin receptor.

Lupus erythematosus

A disease in which the body's immune system attacks its own organs. Also called systemic lupus erythematosus (SLE).

Sickle cell anemia

An inherited anemia that results in red blood cells forming a crescent shape. Sickle cells block small vessels and can result in injury to the bones, heart, lungs, and kidneys.

Atherosclerosis

A disease process that involves deposition of cholesterol in the walls of arteries, causing narrowing of the arteries. This can cause blood to clot, further reducing blood flow.

cally to donate for kidney transplantation have half the number of glomeruli. Over a period of time, the remaining glomeruli enlarge or **hypertrophy** and are able to increase their function.

As we age, out glomeruli normally decrease in number due to scarring. This is a silent process without symptoms and signs, and is often overlooked even by doctors.

4. What can damage the kidneys?

Hundreds of things can damage the kidneys. The most common medical problem that causes damage to the kidneys is uncontrolled **diabetes**. When a diabetic has a high blood glucose, this causes an enlargement of a part of the cell wall of the glomerular capillary filter called the basement membrane. Capillaries and other cells begin to enlarge. This leads to scarring or sclerosis of the glomerulus and results in the glomerulus becoming a damaged filter. Proteins from the blood can leak through the damaged filter and appear in the urine. This leakage can lead to further kidney scarring and damage. High blood pressure can contribute to further glomerular scarring and damage. Kidney problems can also be caused by urinary tract infections, medications, surgical procedures, kidney stones, as well as certain types of cancer. Diseases such as **lupus erythematosus** and **sickle cell anemia** can damage many parts of the body including the kidneys. Smoking and elevated cholesterol can cause hardening of the arteries or **atherosclerosis** to occur in the renal arteries that supply the kidneys with blood. **HIV** infection causes kidney problems in some patients. In many patients, multiple problems have contributed to kidney damage. The earlier we are aware of these problems, the better chance we will have of preventing kidney damage.

5. Can kidney disease be inherited?

Our parents have a tremendous influence upon our future health. We inherit one copy of each of our genes from each parent. The most common form of inherited kidney disease is **autosomal dominant polycystic kidney disease (ADPKD)**. In this disease, we only have to inherit one defective gene from either our father or mother. Most, but not all, people who inherit the gene develop some form of renal disease, which can be mild or severe. The gene causes our kidneys to form multiple cysts that increase in number and size over time. Scientists have found the location of two genes for polycystic kidney disease, one of which is on chromosome 16 called the *APCKD1* gene. This gene accounts for 90% of all cases of ADPKD. It can be diagnosed before birth. Another gene, *APCKD2*, has been found on chromosome 4. Screening for cysts is best done after 30 years of age with a kidney sonogram test, which can detect the cysts. An example of a disease where we need defective genes from both our parents is sickle cell anemia. This genetic disorder is most common in black patients, but can be seen in people of Italian, Indian, Hispanic, and other origins. About 5% of patients with sickle cell anemia will develop severe kidney problems. Diseases such as diabetes, hypertension, systemic lupus erythematosus, and kidney stones are more common in patients with parents who have these disorders. Most importantly, our parents are role models for our own lifestyles and behaviors. If our parents smoke cigarettes, we are much more likely to smoke ourselves. An overweight parent is more likely

The Basics

HIV

The etiologic virus in HIV/AIDS infection. HIV can be transmitted through blood transfusion, intravenous drug use, sexual activity, and through a needle stick. HIV cannot be transmitted during dialysis treatments.

Autosomal dominant polycystic kidney disease (ADPKD)

The most common form of inherited kidney disease. Patients inherit the gene from either parent and many cysts form in the kidneys.

to have overweight children. This being said, we are not our parents. Many people are not affected by their genetic heritage. As medical science improves, new medications for diseases make the prognosis for young people with inherited diseases much better than that of their parents.

6. How do I know I have kidney disease?

Kidney disease sneaks up on us. If we develop chest pain, we immediately think of the heart. Cough, fever, and shortness of breath would cause many of us to seek medical attention for pneumonia. Most patients with kidney disease are asymptomatic in the early stages. Swelling of the legs, high blood pressure, blood in the urine, foaming of the urine, or a family history of kidney disease cause some people to be tested for kidney problems. The search for kidney disease begins with a visit to your doctor. He or she may be a family practitioner, internist, pediatrician, or gynecologist. A detailed history will be taken and a complete physical examination performed. The initial tests to screen for kidney disease include a complete blood count, a **blood urea nitrogen (BUN)**, **serum creatinine**, and **urine analysis**. If all these tests are normal, probably no significant renal disease is present. In diabetic patients, a urine test for **microalbumin** can detect very small amounts of albumen. A positive test can predict who has a high chance of developing kidney disease and who would benefit from early aggressive treatment. Other tests include a 24-hour urine collection for protein and creatinine clearance to accurately measure renal function. A kidney sonogram or sound-wave test is a safe way of looking for blockages of the

Blood urea nitrogen (BUN)

A common blood test used to screen patients for kidney disease. An elevated BUN can indicate decreased kidney function.

Serum creatinine

A blood test used to screen patients for kidney disease. Creatinine is a breakdown product of muscle. When the kidney function is decreased, the kidneys filter less creatinine and the serum creatinine level rises.

Urine analysis

A common screening test that looks for the presence of protein, glucose, and cells in the urine. It can help determine if further tests for kidney disease are indicated.

Microalbumin

A test designed to detect very small elevated amounts of the protein albumin in the urine that are not able to be detected by a routine urine analysis.

kidney due to kidney stones, prostate problems, or cysts of the kidney. If these tests are positive, your doctor may refer you to a kidney specialist. This specialist may be a medical kidney doctor, called a nephrologist, or a urologist, who is a surgeon who specializes in diseases of the kidneys, bladder, and prostate. The specialist has seen many different kinds of kidney problems. He or she can answer many of your questions and may want to obtain further testing to give you a specific diagnosis of the cause of your problem.

Kidney disease sneaks up on us. Most patients with kidney disease are asymptomatic in the early stages.

7. How common is kidney disease?

Kidney disease is becoming more and more common. This is in part due to our increased lifespan. Due to many advances is public health measures as well as medical treatments for heart disease, hypertension, and diabetes, we are living longer and more productive lives. When I began my education in medical school in the 1970s, it was very special to see a patient in the hospital who was 100 years old. Now it is much more common. As we live longer, the chance that we will develop disease processes that will affect our kidneys goes up. It is estimated that in patients in the Medicare system in 2004 over the age of 75 years, one million people had chronic kidney disease. In the 65- to 74-year-old age range, 600,000 people suffered from chronic kidney disease. In 2004 an additional 335,963 people were receiving **dialysis** treatments. The numbers are much higher today (about 500,000 patients) because kidney disease is growing at a rapid rate. This is partly due to the rapid increase of new patients with diabetes. As we become more affluent, we have more choices of both type and quantity of food. We are less likely to walk or to engage in physical

Dialysis

A scientific term for the movement of substances across a membrane by a process called diffusion.

activity. We are getting larger. As our weight increases, we increase our chance of developing diabetes. As a result, the number of diabetics in the population has soared. It is estimated that there are over 21 million diabetics in the United States. Because diabetes is the number one cause of kidney disease in industrialized societies, the number of people with kidney disease is increasing rapidly.

Our awareness of kidney disease is also growing. We are more likely to go to the doctor for a routine checkup than our parents. Once we are at the doctor, there is a good chance that blood and urine tests will be ordered. We are targeting those at high risk for kidney disease for screening. Finally, well-known personalities in the media or sports fields, such as Art Buchwald and Alonzo Mourning, have publicly discussed receiving dialysis treatments and a kidney transplant. We have become more knowledgeable about kidney disease and more willing to discuss it with our family and friends. This communication has led us to a better understanding of kidney disease and the need to take it seriously.

8. Can kidney disease be prevented by diet?

Special diets for the treatment of kidney disease have been available for many years. Before dialysis and modern medications were available, the only available treatment for kidney disease was a special diet. People with kidney disease were placed on low-protein diets in the hope that the progression of kidney disease would be slowed. In addition, intake of salt, potassium, phosphorus, and fluid was restricted. People on these diets could live longer, but the quality of their life was poor. They often became malnourished. In the 1980s, studies were conducted on rats with renal disease. Rats placed on low-protein diets showed a dramatic improvement in their survival compared to rats on high-protein diets. This resulted in a great deal of enthusiasm for protein restriction in the diet. Our normal diet in the United States is heavily weighted toward high-protein foods such as meat, fish, poultry, and milk products. Unfortunately, studies in people on low-protein diets were not as conclusive as the studies in rats. Many doctors still recommend a modest restriction in protein intake in patients with kidney disease.

Many patients believe that cranberry juice can be helpful for kidney disease. This idea comes from the ability of fresh cranberry juice to acidify the urine, which can be helpful in urinary tract infection. Patients with urinary tract infection are treated with antibiotics, which are far superior to cranberry juice. Most people with kidney disease will get no benefit from cranberry juice, but it sure tastes good.

Because so many people with kidney disease suffer from hypertension, it is important to consider a low-salt diet. A low-fat diet is important in people with an elevated cholesterol or triglyceride level because vascular disease occurs often in people with kidney disease. Patients with diabetes require special diets.

There is a great deal of information available in books, in magazines, and on the Internet about diet. Many supplements are available. It is extremely important that professional advice be obtained before going on any diet. Only a health professional can look at your individual case, review your blood tests and medical history, and determine if a particular diet is right for you. Many people have spent years on restrictive diets only to dis-

Advice that is good in general can be the worst advice for a specific person.

cover that the diet has been of no benefit or, worse, harmful to their medical condition. Advice that is good in general can be the worst advice for a specific person.

9. What medications can prevent my kidneys from getting worse?

The first medications proven to delay the progression of kidney disease are a class of medications called **angiotensin-converting enzyme inhibitors** (**Table 1**). Doctors and other medical professionals call them ACE inhibitors for short. These medications work by blocking an enzyme that activates a protein called **angiotensin**. ACE inhibitors decrease blood flow to the glomeruli. This decrease in blood flow will prevent scarring of the glomerulus and surrounding tissues. ACE inhibitors lower blood pressure. They are most often taken once or twice a day. They help prevent hardening of the arteries, or atherosclerosis. ACE inhibitors are also helpful in preventing heart attacks and in the treatment of congestive heart failure.

Angiotensin-converting enzyme inhibitors

A class of medications that is useful in treating high blood pressure, stabilizing kidney disease, and improving patients with congestive heart failure. ACE inhibitors stabilize kidney disease by decreasing the amount of protein in the urine and decreasing the damage done by elevated blood pressure.

Angiotensin

A polypeptide produced in the kidney, which causes blood pressure to rise.

Table 1   Common ACE Inhibitors

Brand Name	Generic Name
Aceon	perindopril erbumine
Altace	ramipril
Capoten	captopril
Lotensin	benazepril hydrochloride
Mavik	trandolapril
Prinivil	lisinopril
Univasc	moexipril hydrochloride
Vasotec	enalapril

ACE inhibitors have three major side effects. Cough can occur in 3% to 8% of patients, depending on the study. The cough goes away when the ACE inhibitor is stopped. Skin rash is an uncommon side effect. More severe allergic reactions causing swelling of the face or lips are uncommon. This is called **angioedema** and must be recognized and treated immediately by your doctor. ACE inhibitors can cause an elevation in the potassium level. Potassium is an element in the blood and body. Too high or too low a potassium level can affect the function of the heart. Blood tests will be needed after you start ACE inhibitor medication and afterward on a regular basis to watch your potassium level. If your potassium level is too high, your doctor or healthcare professional may recommend that you decrease your intake of potassium-rich foods. He or she may place you on a potassium-lowering medication called Kayexalate to bind the potassium in your gastrointestinal tract. If your potassium is still too high, you may be told to stop taking your ACE inhibitor. In rare cases, your kidney function may get worse on ACE inhibitors. This is more common in people who have vascular disease or who are dehydrated. Regular blood tests can help your doctor or healthcare professional identify this problem, which will improve after the ACE inhibitor is stopped.

A second and newer class of medications proven to prevent kidney disease from getting worse is **angiotensin receptor blockers**, or **ARBs (Table 2)**. Like ACE inhibitors, these medications are taken orally, lower blood pressure, and help protect the heart. They can raise potassium, cause rashes, and worsen kidney function but they do not cause cough. Because ARBs are newer med-

Angioedema

A serious allergic reaction characterized by swelling of a body part, often the face or lips.

Angiotensin receptor blockers (ARBs)

A class of medications that has similar properties to ACE inhibitors. ARBs can treat high blood pressure, stabilize kidney disease, decrease protein in the urine, and treat congestive heart failure.

Table 2   Common Angiotensin Receptor Blockers (ARBs)

Brand Name	Generic Name
Atacand	candesartan cilexetil
Avapro	irbesartan
Benicar	olmesartan medoxomil
Cozaar	losartan potassium
Diovan	valsartan
Micardis	telmisartan
Teveten	eprosartan mesylate

ications, they are more expensive; low-cost generic versions of these drugs are just becoming available.

Many advertisements by drug companies encourage the belief that their ACE inhibitor or ARB is better than all the others. They will list multiple advantages and often feature smiling models posing as patients or doctors testifying to the superiority of their medication and low number of side effects. It is too early to tell if ACE inhibitors or ARBs are better. Medical research may help decide this question. Time will tell. Some kidney doctors (nephrologists) will use ACE inhibitors and ARBs together. If this is done, the patient must come for blood tests and frequent visits to prevent complications.

Other medications may be helpful in stabilizing kidney function. Additional medications to control blood pressure and cholesterol are commonly needed. Patients with diabetes must pay special attention to optimize their medication to control their blood sugar level.

10. What alternative medicine treatments are available for kidney disease?

Alternative medicine treatments are very popular topics in the media and often are the first thought when we are confronted with medical illness. The advantage of alternative therapies is that they are thought to be less toxic than conventional medical treatments. They are often derived from plants, fungi, minerals, or other substances found in nature. In reality, the separation of alternative and traditional medicine is an artificial distinction. The first physicians often grew medical herbs in their gardens. In the modern era, cyclosporine, a product of a fungus, revolutionized kidney transplantation. This is almost never mentioned as an alternative treatment. Physicians interested in kidney diseases have been intrigued with omega-3 fatty acids found in fish oils. They have been used to treat high cholesterol as well as a kidney disease called **IgA nephropathy**. We are all looking for the next new miracle drug. Hopefully, this new treatment will be natural, nontoxic, and will have few side effects. Because of the great interest in alternative medical treatments, the US National Institutes of Health established the National Center for Complementary and Alternative Medicine in 1998. This center will be supervising much-needed scientific research on complementary and alternative medical treatments to see which are effective. For more information, their Web site can be located at *http://nccam.nih.gov*.

I am often brought advertisements for vitamins or dietary supplements by patients who are interested in alternative medical treatments. Some of them contain

The Basics

Alternative medicine

A medical discipline that uses natural products and diet to treat medical illness.

IgA nephropathy

A disease of the kidney that often presents with blood and protein in the urine. The immunoglobulin IgA is seen in the kidney on biopsy.

It is best to get expert medical advice from a medical professional who is experienced in working with kidney and dialysis patients before taking vitamins or alternative treatments.

potassium, magnesium, or other substances that may not be safe for that particular individual. It is best to get expert medical advice from a medical professional who is experienced in working with kidney and dialysis patients before taking vitamins or alternative treatments.

11. How can I stabilize my kidney function and stay off dialysis?

Sonograms

Medical tests in which sound waves are used to obtain pictures of organs in the body. A kidney sonogram requires no injections of substances or exposure to radiation. Also known as an ultrasound.

Immunosuppressive therapy

Immunosuppressive therapy works by suppressing the activity of the cells and antibodies of the immune system. In the treatment of some kidney diseases, immunosuppressive medicines are given intravenously or orally to decrease the immune response. Kidney transplant patients also need immunosuppressive medications to prevent rejection of the transplant.

Many patients feel devastated when diagnosed with a kidney disease. Thinking that the problem is hopeless and that one's life is over is very common. In reality, kidney disease has good treatment options at all stages. Treatment is widely available and is not experimental but proven to be effective. The first step is to look for reversible causes of kidney disease. Medications that cause kidney disease need to be stopped. Tests to look for blockages of the kidney such as **sonograms** need to be considered. The accurate diagnosis of the cause of kidney disease by kidney biopsy can determine if the patient is a candidate for **immunosuppressive therapy** with a variety of medications. Immunosuppressive medications that are available include steroids, cyclosporine, cyclophosphamide, and others. In most kidney diseases, ACE inhibitors and ARBs can delay the deterioration of renal function. Diet and control of blood pressure, blood sugar, and cholesterol are all important. In many cases, kidney disease can be stabilized and patients can be managed without renal replacement therapy.

Erick Lucero writes:

I found out I had kidney disease by going to my regular doctor. He found that I had an elevated creatinine level in my blood and high blood pressure. I was referred to a nephrologist. The nephrologist performed a complete physical exam, sent me for a sonogram of the kidneys, and had me collect my urine for 24 hours. After these tests, I went for a kidney biopsy. The biopsy stung for a few seconds but was not that bad. I was told that both my kidneys were diseased by something called focal segmental glomerular sclerosis. This disease was causing scarring of the kidneys and was causing my high blood pressure. I took blood pressure medication and a medication called cyclosporine to help prevent the scarring of my kidneys. I had a scary feeling about my future. I knew that dialysis would take a lot of time and effort. I didn't want to accept that I had a kidney problem. My medications were very expensive. Once, I didn't take my medications for three weeks because I reached my maximum yearly benefit from my insurance and I couldn't afford them. I had to wait until the end of December when the new year started and my insurance would pay for the medication again. It was hard to keep my diet.

Despite my kidney disease, I worked full time. I was often tired and sad. My girlfriend gave me good support. In March of 2006, we got married. She was never put off by my kidney disease and encouraged me. When I was sad, she was sad. My wife became pregnant, and we have a beautiful little girl. My daughter helped take my mind off my problems.

The Basics

It was 2 years from the time I learned that I had kidney disease to the time I started dialysis. I stopped drinking alcohol because I figured that if I had one organ damaged, I needed to keep the rest of my body as healthy as possible. To stay off dialysis you have to stay away from salt and potassium and keep your diet. Take your medications. Try and work with your doctor. The better you are at taking your medications and keeping your diet, the longer you will stay off dialysis.

PART TWO

Dialysis

What is dialysis?

Can children be treated with dialysis?

What will happen if I skip a dialysis treatment?

More . . .

12. What is dialysis?

Dialysis is a scientific term for the movement of substances across a membrane by a process called diffusion. If a great deal of a substance is in one place, some of that substance will tend to move out to where the substance is not present. If we gently add a teaspoon of milk to a cup of tea, the milk will diffuse out with time to all areas of the cup. In dialysis, we add a barrier or membrane between two liquids. On one side of the membrane is a liquid with a high concentration of a substance. On the other side of the membrane is a liquid without that substance. If the membrane has small holes or pores, the substance on one side of the membrane will travel or diffuse across the membrane to the other side until the amount on each side is equal. Dialysis membranes are said to be semipermeable. They allow some small substances to pass through while large substances cannot fit through the holes.

In medical dialysis treatments, one liquid is a patient's blood. On the other side of the semipermeable membrane, is another liquid called **dialysate**. Substances in the blood, if they are small enough, will move through the membrane into the dialysate. If the dialysate is then discarded and new dialysate is added, more of the substance can be removed. Removal of substances depends on the size of the substance, the electrical charge of the substance, and also the difference in the amount of the substance on one side of the membrane compared to the other.

If we change the amount of substances in the dialysate, we can remove more or less of a substance. We can even add more of a substance to the dialysate than is in the blood. In this instance, the substance will move

Dialysate

A fluid containing sodium, calcium, bicarbonate, and other substances that is used to remove toxins and poisons during dialysis. Different dialysate solutions are used in hemodialysis and peritoneal dialysis.

from the dialysate into the patient's blood. This can be done with substances that can pass through the semipermeable membrane. If we put a high concentration of the sugar glucose in the dialysate, it will move or diffuse across the membrane into the blood and raise the level of glucose in the blood.

Dialysis sounds complicated, but it all boils down to the process of diffusion. Large things such as red blood cells, large proteins, and other large substances are trapped on one side of the membrane in the blood. Small things including salts such as sodium and potassium, water, and small proteins can freely move across the membrane from areas where large amounts are present to areas where they are not present.

13. When was dialysis invented?

The first time dialysis is mentioned in scientific literature was by Thomas Graham, a Scottish chemist, who wrote about dialysis in 1854. He used an ox bladder for his membrane. George Haas, working in Germany in the 1920s, was the first person to use dialysis to treat patients. Most kidney doctors consider Dr. Willem J. Kolff to be the father of modern dialysis. Working in the Netherlands during World War II, Dr. Kolff was caring for war casualties who were dying of kidney failure. He decided to design and build an artificial kidney. Because medical supplies were limited, he obtained his membrane for dialysis from a sausage factory. This sausage skin was made of cellulose acetate. He also used an automobile water pump in his machine. Dr. Kolff was able to treat a 68-year-old woman with kidney failure and maintain her on dialysis until her own kidneys recovered. Dr. Kolff's creativity in building his equipment during wartime, his success in the treatment of the first patient, and his work as a teacher make him a legend and an inspiration to generations of kidney doctors.

14. What is hemodialysis?

Hemodialysis is a medical treatment in which dialysis is used to remove poisons and toxins from a patient's blood. Blood is obtained from the patient with needles and plastic tubing. The blood is then pumped past a semipermeable dialysis membrane. Poisons and toxins that are usually removed by the kidneys pass through the membrane by diffusion into a liquid called dialysate. The dialysate is then discarded along with the toxins. The purified blood is then returned to the patient's body.

Because the patient's blood is outside of the body, a modern dialysis machine has a warmer to keep the blood at body temperature. A blood thinner called **heparin** is given to prevent the blood from clotting in the plastic tubing or when in contact with the dialysis membrane. The hemodialysis machine has safety equipment to determine if the hemodialysis is going well (**Figure 3**). These sensors may sound an alarm to help guide the staff. These alarms do not signify danger to the patient. The modern hemodialysis machine has benefitted greatly from the computer age. The electronic chips and integrated circuits in the dialysis machine make dialysis accurate, safe, and reliable. This has improved the quality of care.

Hemodialysis

A medical treatment in which blood is removed from the patient with needles and plastic tubing and pumped past the dialysis membrane. Poisons and toxins cross the dialysis membrane into the dialysate, which is then discarded, and the blood is returned to the patient.

Heparin

An acid that occurs naturally in the liver and lungs that can be purified and used as a medication to prevent blood from clotting. Heparin is used in hemodialysis to prevent blood from clotting in the plastic tubing and when exposed to the dialysis membrane. It can also be injected into the peritoneal dialysis fluid to prevent clots from blocking the peritoneal dialysis catheter.

Dialysis

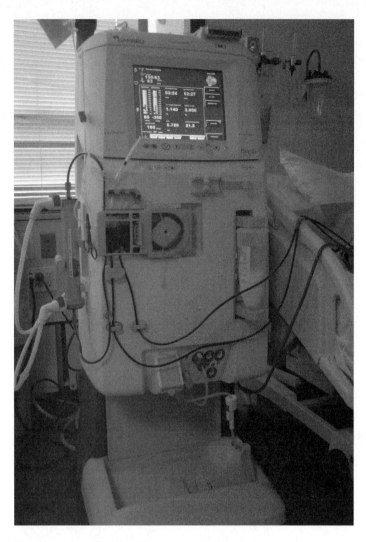

> *The modern hemodialysis machine has benefitted greatly from the computer age. The electronic chips and integrated circuits in the dialysis machine make dialysis accurate, safe, and reliable.*

Figure 3   A hemodialysis machine
Source: K. Neelakantappa, MD

15. What is peritoneal dialysis?

Peritoneal dialysis is a type of dialysis in which a patient's peritoneum is used as the dialysis membrane. The peritoneum is a membrane that covers our intestines inside our abdomen. It is a naturally occurring

Peritoneal dialysis

Dialysis treatments that use the patient's peritoneal membrane in the abdomen as a dialysis membrane to remove toxins and wastes from the body.

membrane. In hemodialysis, an artificial membrane is used. In peritoneal dialysis, we take advantage of the semipermeable qualities of a naturally occurring membrane.

In peritoneal dialysis, a permanent flexible plastic tube is inserted into the abdomen by a physician. This tube is called the peritoneal dialysis catheter. After the tissues around the tube have healed, the tube is used to instill dialysate into the abdomen. The dialysate fluid is allowed to remain in the abdomen for several hours. During this time, poisons and toxins leave the blood vessels of the intestine, pass through the peritoneal membrane, and collect in the dialysate fluid. The dialysate is then drained by gravity through the peritoneal dialysis catheter and collected in a bag. The dialysate fluid containing poisons and toxins can then be discarded into a sink drain or toilet. Another bag of dialysate, usually containing 2 liters of fluid is then infused into the abdomen. Each dialysis drainage and infusion is called an exchange because the fluid is removed and replaced. Patients usually perform four exchanges every day.

The peritoneal dialysis exchanges are initially done by the peritoneal dialysis nurse. The patient on peritoneal dialysis is then trained over a period of weeks to safely perform the dialysis. The exchanges can be done at home, at work, or in any clean, quiet place because no special machine is required. This form of peritoneal dialysis is called **continuous ambulatory peritoneal dialysis**, or **CAPD**. The continuous means that the dialysis will continue throughout the day. Ambulatory refers to the dialysis being done outside of a hospital or medical facility. CAPD is the most popular form of peritoneal dialysis. It is usually done by the person on

Continuous ambulatory peritoneal dialysis (CAPD)

A home dialysis procedure taught to patients who perform their own peritoneal dialysis, CAPD involves the instillation by gravity of dialysate through a catheter into the abdomen. The fluid remains in the abdomen for a time, allowing poisons and toxins to accumulate in the dialysate. The dialysate is then drained and discarded, and fresh dialysate is instilled.

dialysis, but it can also be done by other family members. In the case of children on dialysis, the parents usually perform the dialysis. Elderly patients with many health problems can also have family members perform dialysis. Peritoneal dialysis can also be done at night with the aid of a machine called a **cycler**. This machine is set up before sleep in the patient's bedroom at home. It will then automatically perform the exchanges during the night. This form of peritoneal dialysis is called **continuous cyclical peritoneal dialysis**, or **CCPD**. It allows the patient to be free during the day to work or go to school without performing their exchanges. Family members can also set up the cycler at night without interfering with their daytime activities. Peritoneal dialysis done in a dialysis center is not common but is available in a few dialysis units.

Cycler

A machine used to automate peritoneal dialysis by performing the exchange of peritoneal dialysis fluid.

Continuous cyclical peritoneal dialysis (CPPD)

A home peritoneal dialysis procedure that uses a cycler to instill and drain fluid into the abdomen. The cycler can perform peritoneal dialysis while the patient is sleeping.

16. Which treatment will be best for me, hemodialysis, peritoneal dialysis, or a kidney transplant?

When faced with kidney disease and the need for renal replacement therapy, most people are overwhelmed. It is difficult to decide which therapy is best. Initially, most patients are treated with hemodialysis at a dialysis center. At the hemodialysis center, the dialysis is performed by the dialysis staff. This allows the patient to get used to the hemodialysis treatment, learn about their diet and medications, and grow stronger. The adjustment to dialysis is both physical and emotional. The dialysis staff will help with this adjustment. Other patients in the dialysis center are able to provide support and advice because they have had to cope with a similar adjustment in the past. Hemodialysis is safe, effective, and well tolerated by most patients. Patients are usually treated three times a week at the same time on Monday, Wednesday, Friday or on Tuesday, Thursday, Saturday. Most dialysis units are closed on Sunday. Treatments are organized in shifts with many patients beginning and ending at about the same time. Patients have 4 days when they do not have hemodialysis treatments. They, however, must keep their diet and take medication 7 days a week.

Patients on peritoneal dialysis start their treatments at a peritoneal dialysis center or unit. The dialysis staff begins the treatment and trains the patients to perform their own dialysis treatment. This training takes several weeks. Most people can learn how to perform the peritoneal dialysis exchanges. Patients usually require 4 exchanges a day, 7 days a week. Because peritoneal dialysis is done 7 days a week, fluid and poisons are removed continuously every day. This continuous treatment allows an increased intake of fluid and a more varied diet. Hemodialysis treatments are typically three times a week. Between hemodialysis treatments, fluid, potassium, salt, and phosphorus intake must be limited. Another advantage of peritoneal dialysis is the ability to vary your dialysis schedule by changing the time or the location of your exchanges. Peritoneal dialysis allows greater flexibility of travel because there is no need to be in a dialysis center or to have a dialysis machine.

Kidney transplantation is a very attractive option for renal replacement therapy because no dialysis is needed. A kidney transplant can come from a family member, a person who is not a blood relative like a spouse or a friend, or from a donor who has died. Most patients need to be treated with some form of dialysis before a kidney transplant can be accomplished. Sometimes a transplant is done before dialysis is needed. Kidney transplant patients must take immunosuppressive medication to prevent rejection of the kidney transplant for as long as the transplant is working.

We are very fortunate to have three good treatments for renal replacement therapy. Many patients start on hemodialysis as an initial therapy. As they become more knowledgeable, they may switch to peritoneal dialysis when they feel capable of performing their own dialysis treatments. Some patients learn to perform home hemodialysis that also requires special training. Many patients on dialysis plan to receive a kidney transplant. Others prefer to remain on dialysis. Transplant recipients facing loss of their transplant from rejection can choose to return to hemodialysis or peritoneal dialysis.

We are very fortunate to have three good treatments for renal replacement therapy.

It is very likely that patients with kidney failure will be treated with more than one kind of treatment modality during their lifetime. The choice of the initial therapy is less important than we tend to think. If we are unhappy with our choice or experience difficulties with one therapy, we can change to another renal replacement therapy.

17. Can children be treated with dialysis?

Children can be treated with hemodialysis or peritoneal dialysis. Between 1995 and 2004, over 7,000 children required renal replacement therapy in the United States. As in adult patients, more children are begun on hemodialysis than on peritoneal dialysis. Kidney transplantation is the preferred treatment in children. This is because children's physical growth is less than normal on dialysis. Three out of four children on dialysis receive a transplant within three years. Transplantation offers the best hope for normal growth and development as well as enabling children to participate in school and athletics. The availability of parents as healthy potential donors makes transplantation a good option. Siblings must be over 18 years of age to donate a kidney.

18. Where will I go for dialysis?

In the early days of dialysis, dialysis units were at major medical centers. As the need for dialysis has grown, many more units have opened. Dialysis has become safer and routine. Instead of being in a hospital, most units are now freestanding. This means they are in the community closer to home. Your dialysis unit may be in a shopping center, may be a separate building, or may be part of an office building. Many of us pass these units every day unaware of their existence. When you walk into a dialysis unit, you will enter a reception area or waiting room. Nearby is the treatment area, which is a large room containing 10 to 20 dialysis stations. Each dialysis station has a dialysis machine, a reclining chair, and usually an individual television set. Many dialysis units have computers for record keeping. The stations are in a line to be easily visible to the dialysis staff. There is a central nursing station with telephones, medications, and other equipment. Close to the treatment area but not visible to patients are rooms to purify water, make dialysate, and service equipment.

More dialysis units have opened in suburban and rural locations. Patients living in a high population area such as a city often have several units close by from which to choose. Units in cities are large, with many able to dialyze 20 or more patients on each dialysis shift. Rural units are smaller and farther apart. When dialysis started, most units were owned by hospitals, single individuals, or not-for-profit organizations. In the 1980s ownership of dialysis units changed. Units owned by hospitals, individuals, and not-for-profit foundations remained about the same. Units run by large chains began to grow. These chains are owned by large public corporations. Some of these corporations also manufacture dialysis machines or equipment. The large size of these chains has enabled them to take advantage of buying larger quantities of supplies and equipment at a lower price, and enabled them to open large numbers of units. The highest concentration of dialysis units is in the eastern half of the country. Areas along the Gulf coast and eastern seaboard have many more units than in the western portion of the United States. How long you need to travel to the dialysis unit will influence your choice of therapy. If it takes you several hours to reach the nearest unit, home dialysis or transplantation would be a definite advantage. Most home dialysis and transplant patients when they are stable visit the dialysis unit or doctor's office once a month for evaluation.

19. Who will perform my dialysis treatments?

With in-center hemodialysis, the dialysis staff will perform your dialysis. The role of the physician is to evaluate the patient, determine the specifics of the dialysis treatment, write dialysis orders, and be available for problems and questions. Other staff include **registered nurses**, **licensed practical nurses**, and

Registered nurse

A healthcare professional who has graduated from a nursing program and passed state qualifying examinations.

Licensed practical nurse

A healthcare professional who has completed a nursing program and passed a licensing exam. An LPN works under the supervision of registered nurses and physicians.

Dialysis technician

A healthcare worker who works in the hemodialysis unit under the supervision of a registered nurse. Dialysis technicians can institute hemodialysis by inserting needles into the access, and can also monitor the dialysis treatment, measure blood pressure, and help educate dialysis patients regarding their treatment, but they are not allowed to administer medication.

Nurse practitioner

A nurse who has received additional training in the diagnosis and treatment of diseases. The nurse practitioner is able to prescribe medication and perform medical procedures.

Physician assistant

A member of the healthcare team who works under the supervision of a physician and diagnoses and manages medical problems.

dialysis technicians. State law determines who can perform which functions in the dialysis unit. In most states, the administration of medications is done by registered nurses. The nurses and technicians connect the patient to the machine and monitor the dialysis treatment. Some units have **nurse practitioners** and **physician assistants** as part of the dialysis staff. **Dietitians** and **social workers** are important members of the dialysis team. Dialysis units have a large support staff. Technicians maintain and service equipment. Housekeeping chores such as taking out the garbage and mopping the floors never end. The clerical staff records treatments, orders supplies, and helps submit insurance claims.

Patients on peritoneal dialysis perform their own dialysis treatments. At first, they will perform their dialysis under the supervision of the dialysis nurse. As the patients become more skilled and comfortable with their dialysis, they will be able to perform it alone without help. This adjustment may take 1 to 2 weeks. They will still need to be carefully followed until they are fully comfortable with the peritoneal dialysis procedure. Patients are also taught to self-administer medications. When the training has been completed, they need to come to the dialysis unit once a month for evaluation by the peritoneal dialysis nurse and physician. The patient is examined by the nurse and physician. Blood tests are obtained every month to monitor the dialysis, and changes in the dialysis prescription may be made. Home hemodialysis patients usually come to the dialysis unit every month. Home visits are useful to help optimize the dialysis treatments.

20. Who will be on dialysis with me at the dialysis center?

Patients on dialysis will reflect the composition of the community in which the unit is located. Most of us do not want to travel to receive health care. We may be willing to travel to see a specialist or to have a complicated procedure or operation. Once we are stable and our lives are back to normal, convenience is much more important. Patients on hemodialysis will come to the dialysis center three times a week. If we are able to go to a center close to our home, we will have more time to spend with family or for recreation, or we will be able to keep working at our job. If a problem arises, it is easier to come in to the dialysis unit to be evaluated by the nursing or medical staff. Rain, snow, storms, tornados, hurricanes are less of a problem if our travel to dialysis is short.

Since 1980, patients aged 45 to 64 years have accounted for about 40% of the patients on dialysis. This statistic is due to the aging of the baby boom generation. The median age of patients on dialysis is 64.8 years. There are few patients younger than 18 and older than 90 years of age. As people live longer and dialysis treatments improve, older patients are now being offered treatment with dialysis. More men are on dialysis than women, with a ratio of 1.2 to 1. More patients live in urban than rural areas. Sixty-six percent of patients are white, 30% are black, 3.5% are Asian, and 1% are Native Americans. Culturally, the number of Hispanic patients is growing, as is the Hispanic population of the United States.

Dietitian

A registered health professional who has special training in nutrition. Dietitians advise patients on which foods to eat and which to avoid based upon their individual needs. They use monthly laboratory tests to monitor the patient's progress.

Social worker

A licensed professional who is part of the multidisciplinary team at the dialysis unit. The social worker assists patients with emotional, financial, and social issues and also provides education and referrals to community resources. A nephrology social worker specializes in services that support patients and families who are adjusting to the major lifestyle changes that are caused by end stage renal disease.

Dialysis

A dialysis unit is a microcosm of society. Patients are from all ethnic groups, occupations, religions, and economic backgrounds.

Patients with diabetes as the primary cause of their renal failure account for about 45% of patients on dialysis. The second largest group of patients has hypertension, but the hypertension may be due to many different causes. Other common causes of renal failure are glomerulonephritis and cystic kidney diseases. A dialysis unit is a microcosm of society. Patients are from all ethnic groups, occupations, religions, and economic backgrounds.

21. Who will pay for my dialysis treatments?

Dialysis treatments are expensive. In-center hemodialysis costs about $40,000 to $50,000 a year. Home hemodialysis or peritoneal dialysis is less costly because the person on dialysis performs the treatment.

In 1972, the United States Congress became concerned that the high cost of dialysis was limiting patients' ability to receive treatment. They amended the Social Security Act, making kidney dialysis patients eligible for **Medicare** regardless of their age. This enabled large numbers of patients to receive dialysis treatments, and led to the rapid growth in the number of dialysis units. Patients can qualify for Medicare by working long enough to be insured under Social Security or under other programs such as the Railroad Retirement Board. You may also receive Medicare if you are the husband, wife, or child (under 18 years of age) of someone who has worked long enough to qualify for Social Security. You may also be eligible for Medicare based upon a disability before you need dialysis treatments.

Medicare will pay for 80% of the cost of dialysis treatment including medications given during the

Medicare

A federally-funded program that provides medical treatments and services to patients over the age of 65 and to patients who are younger than 65 and disabled.

dialysis treatment. It will also pay 80% of the costs of hospitalization, x-rays, and doctor fees. Medicare has two parts, A and B. In order to have part B coverage, a premium must be paid of about $92 a month. More information regarding Medicare can be obtained by calling the Medicare Patient Hotline at 800-442-2620, or by visiting the Medicare Web site at *www.medicare.gov.*

Many private insurances cover some or all of the costs of dialysis treatments. If your insurance covers 80% of the cost, you can be eligible for Medicare to pay the remaining 20%. After 30 months, Medicare will become the primary insurance, paying 80%, and your private insurance will pay the remaining 20%.

Recently, many people have enrolled in health maintenance organizations, or HMOs, to provide for their health insurance. Many HMOs have conditions limiting the dialysis unit in which you can obtain treatment. If this happens, it is important to ask the HMO and your dialysis unit to try to obtain approval for your treatment.

Patients without health insurance may be eligible for the **Medicaid** program. Medicaid is administered by the individual states. Eligibility may be different for patients requiring dialysis treatments than for other patients. Patients who are not United States citizens can also be covered under the Medicaid program.

By now, you are probably totally confused and discouraged by how complicated paying for dialysis treatments seems. You are not alone. Most patients are overwhelmed by the rules and regulations for health insurance. The high cost of dialysis treatments makes

Medicaid

A federally-funded insurance program that is administered by the states to provide medical services, medications, and transportatlon to medical treatments for patients who have limited monetary resources.

this issue even more anxiety producing. Fortunately, no one is denied dialysis treatments in the United States based on their inability to pay. All dialysis units have dedicated social workers and other staff who are experts in the insurance process and who are available to guide you with these issues.

22. I have heard that dialysis is painful. Is this true?

I often tell people considering dialysis treatments that the worst part of dialysis is thinking about it! Our imaginations are always worse than reality. It is important when considering dialysis treatments to visit a dialysis center, observe treatments, and talk to people actually undergoing treatment.

Access

A device that is inserted or constructed in a patient which connects the patient to the dialysis tubing and allows dialysis to take place. In hemodialysis, an access allows blood to be drawn and can be an arterial-venous (a-v) fistula, a-v graft, or a dialysis catheter. The access for peritoneal dialysis (the peritoneal dialysis catheter) is a plastic tube that allows dialysate to be instilled into the abdomen.

In the pre-dialysis period, an **access** must be created before dialysis can be performed. In hemodialysis, a small tube is constructed in the arm between an artery and a vein. This tube allows needles to be inserted to obtain blood for the dialysis treatment. A plastic tube or catheter may be inserted in the blood vessels in the neck to obtain blood. In peritoneal dialysis, a plastic tube is inserted in the abdomen to instill the dialysis fluid. The creation of these accesses are minor surgical procedures. They are associated with mild to moderate pain that usually is treated with oral pain medications such as Tylenol (acetaminophen), Tylenol with codeine, or similar medications until the pain goes away in a day or two.

The most physically painful part of hemodialysis is the insertion of needles in the access in the arm for obtaining blood for the dialysis treatment. Some patients use an anesthetic spray. Most patients on hemodialysis rapidly get used to having needles inserted. Occasionally, muscle cramps in the arms or legs may occur during treatment when too much fluid is being removed. If you have a cramp, telling the dialysis staff will allow them to stop removing fluid or even to give some fluid back. Massaging the affected muscle can also help. Hemodialysis requires sitting in a reclining chair for about 4 hours of treatment. This can be difficult for some people. If you have arthritis or other chronic painful conditions, it is important to consider taking medication for pain before your treatment. Patients come to dialysis with their favorite travel pillow, blanket, book, iPod, or DVD player to make the treatment more comfortable.

Patients on peritoneal dialysis can have abdominal pain, which is often a sign of infection or peritonitis. It is important that patients recognize this and seek help from their dialysis center for evaluation and treatment.

Beginning dialysis is often psychologically painful. We are concerned about the effect dialysis treatments will have on our lives, loved ones, and our future health. Our sense of "well-being" is shaken. These feelings are often accompanied by depression. All these thoughts and feelings are perfectly normal. It is important to express these thoughts to the dialysis staff as well as your physician. They are specially trained to support people beginning dialysis. Remember, they have seen hundreds of people begin and cope with dialysis. You are beginning dialysis for the first time.

One of my patients, who I will call George, suffers from congenital deafness. Because of high blood pressure and diabetes, he was forced to consider dialysis treatments at age 50. After a great deal of resistance to beginning treatment, he ended up in the hospital and began hemodialysis. After a year, during one of our team meetings, he told me that we should change the name of the dialysis center to the dialysis spa. He said that for him, the idea of dialysis as a medical treatment was too negative and depressing. The idea of a spa treatment, away from the demands and frustrations of everyday life, made dialysis less painful for him. He emphasized that the time on dialysis allowed him to think, rest, and read without interruption.

When you visit a dialysis center before beginning your dialysis treatment, ask patients how they cope with their treatment. Most patients will be glad to talk to you.

Many of my patients cope with dialysis treatments by considering dialysis to be a part-time job. Work for them is a source of pride, something that is difficult but, with effort, can be accomplished. There are as many coping mechanisms as there are patients on dialysis. When you visit a dialysis center before beginning your dialysis treatment, ask patients how they cope with their treatment. Most patients will be glad to talk to you. They will remember beginning dialysis and their own fears and misconceptions. This will help you develop your own strategy that is right for you.

Erick Lucero writes:

When I first started dialysis, I had a catheter inserted by a surgeon. The next procedure I had was an a-v (arterial-venous) fistula in my right arm near my wrist. Dialysis using the catheter was not painful. Instead of using needles, there are small caps on the catheter that are unscrewed, and the catheter is connected to the hemodialysis tubing. When it was time to use my fistula after 3 months, the needles were inserted. This was very painful at first. I got used to the needles with time. They still hurt, but the pain lasts for a very short time.

The other painful parts of dialysis are the cramps I get in my legs when too much fluid is removed. I can take off two and a half liters during my treatment. If I try to take off three liters, I sometimes get severe cramps in my calves. This usually lasts 5 minutes. You have to know your body on dialysis and how much fluid you can take off without having cramps.

23. What will happen if I skip a dialysis treatment?

Most people on dialysis are confronted with obligations and commitments that interfere with dialysis treatments. A child might be sick. A favorite niece may have a wedding on a dialysis day. A bad cold may make us reluctant to leave the house. Things happen at inconvenient times. Bad weather may make travel to the dialysis unit difficult or impossible. Very rarely, power outages or problems with the water supply may make it impossible for a dialysis center to treat patients for a short period of time.

In most instances, missing or postponing a single hemodialysis treatment does not result in a catastrophe. If patients are having effective dialysis treatments, adhering to their diet and fluid restrictions, and taking their medications properly, dialysis can be rescheduled for later the same day or even the next day safely. Patients who are not receiving good dialysis or keeping their diet may develop puffiness around the face, fluid in the legs, and shortness of breath. This is due to fluid overload. Typically, these symptoms occur on Sunday or Monday night because of the longer interval between hemodialysis treatments on those days. Often,

Peripheral nervous system

Nerves that leave the spinal cord and go to the organs, muscles, and skin. These nerves carry information from the brain to the body, and also bring information back to the brain.

Uremic neuropathy

Damage to nerves that is caused by the toxins and poisons that build up in the blood in kidney failure. Typical symptoms of uremic neuropathy are tingling or numbness in the feet and hands. Uremic neuropathy is treated by increasing the amount of dialysis that the patient is receiving to remove the build-up of toxins and poisons. Medications are sometimes used to treat the symptoms of uremic neuropathy.

High-flux dialysis

A procedure that uses high blood flows and large dialysis membranes to remove poisons and toxins in a shorter dialysis treatment, although short dialysis treatments are no longer recommended. The experience with high flux dialysis helped kidney doctors improve dialysis treatments by removing more toxins during regular hemodialysis treatments.

patients tend to go off their diets on weekends due to parties or other social occasions.

Dialysis is a renal replacement therapy. Our own kidneys work 24 hours a day, 7 days a week. Dialysis does not replace all of our renal function. Hemodialysis 3 times a week at best replaces 12% to 15% of normal renal function. If we miss one hemodialysis treatment, we miss one-third of our weekly renal replacement therapy. This can result in immediate problems such as too much fluid in our body or a high potassium level in our blood. Weakness, fatigue, and loss of appetite can occur. If dialysis treatments are missed frequently, the toxins and poisons that build up in our blood can damage our **peripheral nervous system**. This is called **uremic neuropathy**. Symptoms include numbness and tingling of the hands and feet, pain, and weakness. The poisons can cause inflammation in the lining of our heart, or pericarditis. Fluid overload from missing many treatments can put a strain on the heart, leading to an enlarged heart that is not able to effectively pump blood. Poisons can affect the lining of our stomach and cause gastritis, which in turn can cause decreased appetite, abdominal pain, nausea, and vomiting. In severe forms, bleeding can occur, which may require admission to a hospital for emergency treatment.

Many patients ask if they can be treated with one or two hemodialysis treatments a week. In the 1980s, physicians tried to decrease the time spent on hemodialysis with treatments called **high-flux dialysis**. These approaches resulted in more complications and a shortened life span in patients on dialysis. Scientific experts now recommend that we increase the amount of dialysis treatment to prevent complications and improve the quality and length of life.

Patients on peritoneal dialysis are fortunate that they can adjust the timing of their treatment. Then can perform their exchanges at times that are convenient because they are not dependent on the dialysis center schedule. The peritoneal dialysis staff can guide you on the proper spacing of exchanges. Peritoneal dialysis patients must be self-motivated. If they fail to perform one of their daily exchanges, no one will remind them. If an in-center hemodialysis patient fails to come for treatment, usually a dialysis staff member will call the person to ask why he or she missed a treatment and try to reschedule the treatment. Patients on home hemodialysis can also vary the time of their treatments to fit their schedule. Home dialysis is often a good choice for people with busy careers who may have to adjust their schedules.

Most long-time survivors on dialysis have certain characteristics. First, they accept the need for their treatments both intellectually and emotionally. They participate in the planning of their treatments and understand the factors that result in a successful treatment. These long-term survivors take the necessary steps to ensure that they receive a better treatment and resist the temptation to cut their treatment. Secondly, these patients engage in a healthy lifestyle. They keep their diet, avoid excess alcohol, abstain from smoking, try to exercise. Thirdly, they are very careful to take their medications correctly. If they have hypertension or diabetes, they control these conditions with diet and medication. By accomplishing these things, they avoid many of the complications for renal failure that interfere with quality of life and longevity. Achieving these goals takes time, and most people are not perfect. By developing good habits when beginning dialysis, a routine can be established that can promote health and effective treatment for renal failure.

24. Now that I am on dialysis, can I eat whatever I want?

Before beginning dialysis, patients are often on very restrictive diets to delay the need for dialysis. As kidney disease progresses, the kidneys have a harder time eliminating fluid, and salts, such as potassium and sodium, from the body. Often, diuretics are prescribed to increase the urine output and the excretion of fluid, sodium, and potassium. Eating less sodium, potassium, phosphorus, and fluid compensates for a decreased ability to get rid of these substances. In the early days in the development of dialysis, a limited number of dialysis facilities resulted in many patients delaying dialysis and becoming increasingly debilitated and malnourished. Patients were often placed on low-protein diets and lost part of their muscle mass. They would begin dialysis in a debilitated state and require months of rehabilitation and nutritional support to get back to a state of good health. Now we know that it is better to begin dialysis before these nutritional changes occur and try to preserve muscle mass and nutritional reserves.

An individual's nutritional needs will vary greatly, and it is very important to get expert advice from a registered dietitian who has experience with dialysis patients. This individual evaluation is much more important for kidney patients than for patients with other medical conditions. Every dialysis center has dietary specialists who can take a dietary history and, in consultation with your doctor, develop a diet that is optimized for you.

What you should eat will depend on many factors. Underlying medical problems such as diabetes, elevated cholesterol, and lactose intolerance are just a few examples of conditions that will affect what you eat. Men and women have different dietary needs. Body size and activity level also determine your nutritional needs. The type of dialysis that you choose will also determine your diet. Some patients continue to make urine and have residual renal function. The kidneys are excreting some salt, fluid, and toxins that allow the patient to ingest an additional amount of fluid equal to this urine output.

Hemodialysis three times a week is the most common dialysis therapy. Because this treatment is intermittent, fluid potassium, sodium, and phosphorus, all increase in the body between dialysis treatments. During a 4-hour treatment, an average of 2 liters of fluid is removed. Fluid will then accumulate in your body until the next treatment. The amount of fluid you can safely consume between treatments will include the fluid you excrete in the urine as well as fluid excreted by the lungs and in stool. The goal is to prevent the need for the removal of large amounts of fluid in a short time. If it is necessary to remove a great deal of fluid, complications during dialysis such as muscle cramps, a fall in blood pressure, and dizziness after treatments can occur. Potassium and salt will also have to be restricted in the diet to prevent them from building up in the body. Protein intake is usually recommended to be 1 to 1.2 grams per kilogram of body weight. Many dietitians have food models to give patients an idea of portion size that is included in their diet. They can also try to incorporate patients' favorite foods into their dietary plan.

In peritoneal dialysis, treatment occurs on a continuous basis every day, enabling the patient to ingest an increased amount of fluid. The treatment can be

An individual's nutritional needs will vary greatly, and it is very important to get expert advice from a registered dietitian who has experience with dialysis patients.

Dialysis

adjusted to remove more or less fluid by varying the dextrose or sugar content of the peritoneal dialysis solutions. If we wish to remove more fluid, a higher dextrose-containing solution will osmotically pull out more fluid from the body. This will enable patients to drink more in the course of the day. Patients may also eat more potassium on peritoneal dialysis. Protein can be excreted in peritoneal dialysis because it can pass through the peritoneal dialysis membrane. It is important to take this into consideration and continue to consume enough protein in your diet.

The role of diet is probably the most underestimated factor affecting the health of patients. The more we learn of the science of nutrition as patients and healthcare professionals, the better prepared we will be to achieve good outcomes on dialysis.

25. What medicines are removed by my dialysis treatments?

We think of dialysis as a life-saving procedure that removes dangerous poisons and toxins from our blood and our bodies. Dialysis will also remove substances that are beneficial and healthy for us. Examples of these substances are vitamins and medications. As long as a substance can be dissolved in water (water-soluble), and it is not too large, there is a good chance that it will pass from the blood through the dialysis membrane into the dialysate. Hemodialysis and peritoneal dialysis membranes are different and have different clearances. Insulin, a protein, can easily pass through the peritoneal dialysis membrane but cannot pass through the hemodialysis membrane. Many of the water soluble vitamins such as vitamin C, folate, and the B vitamins are removed during hemodialysis and peritoneal dialysis, which is why many dialysis patients are placed on vitamin supplements. If you eat a healthy, varied diet containing fruits and vegetables, this loss is not significant.

Some antibiotics such as penicillin and ampicillin are removed by dialysis. In general, when taking antibiotics, it is wise to take your dose after your dialysis treatment. This will decrease the amount of medication removed by your treatment. Seizure medicines such as phenytoin are also removed by hemodialysis. It is important for your doctor to check blood levels to guide you on the proper dose of this medicine. Other medications removed by dialysis include aspirin and lithium. In fact, overdoses of some medications are sometimes treated with hemodialysis. Alcohol readily passes through the dialysis membrane.

26. Will I be able to keep my job after beginning dialysis?

Work is an important part of our lives. We often define ourselves by what we do. We are a police officer, farmer, engineer, teacher, secretary, or carpenter. In addition to our salary, we have the benefits of feeling useful to others, camaraderie with fellow workers, and the self-esteem of a job well done. We rely on our jobs for financial security and often for health insurance.

Most people plan to take time off from work when starting dialysis. Beginning dialysis treatments is stressful. You may find that it is difficult to concentrate on work and risk performing poorly. Every occupation is different, some more stressful and demanding than others. How much time you take off from work depends on several factors. Patients who delay beginning dialysis for a long time may feel weak and debilitated. They may eat poorly and lose muscle mass. Their ability to perform tasks at work may decrease. Dialysis patients who also have other medical conditions such as heart problems, recent surgery, and poor nutritional status may need a longer adjustment period. Every job is different. The level of physical activity, amount of time at work, and travel for work all are important considerations.

Most people plan to take time off from work when starting dialysis. Beginning dialysis treatments is stressful.

I tell my patients they should try to take off a minimum of at least 2 weeks while adjusting to dialysis. During the second week, they can review their progress with the dialysis team and begin to plan their return to work. Many patients go back to work part time at first. This allows them to rest more and decreases the stress associated with starting dialysis.

Peritoneal dialysis patients will have to decide on the timing of their peritoneal dialysis exchanges. Most people will perform one exchange at home before going to work, one exchange during their lunch period, one exchange when returning home, and one before bedtime. It is possible to be on peritoneal dialysis at night by using a machine called a cycler. You can set the machine up at home, and it will complete your exchanges automatically while you sleep. In the morning, you can disconnect from the machine and have no dialysis during the day, allowing your full attention to be devoted to work. Peritoneal and home dialysis can help by eliminating your travel time to the dialysis unit. Many patients on hemodialysis can use their time on hemodialysis to be productive. The modern laptop computer can allow highly motivated and accomplished patients to write letters, answer e-mail, and research presentations all while receiving dialysis treatment. Other patients prefer their dialysis treatment time to be work free and would rather watch television, read, or sleep on dialysis. Certainly, you should not depend upon working while receiving dialysis. Episodes of low blood pressure, machine alarms, and the measuring of vital signs including heart rate and blood pressure every 15 to 30 minutes by the dialysis staff may make the idea of working on hemodialysis overly optimistic for many patients.

Some patients beginning dialysis choose to change their careers. They use the first year or two on dialysis to go to school and retrain in a profession that is more compatible with their dialysis lifestyle. Chronic renal failure is sometimes grounds for being placed on disability. Your dialysis team, especially the social worker, will be able to help you determine if you meet the criteria for disability in your state.

Erick Lucero writes:

My doctor and I were working hard to save my kidney function. I was on a medication called cyclosporine that I hoped would stabilize my kidney function and prevent the need for dialysis. Suddenly my blood tests were worse and my potassium was high. I received a call from my doctor on June 1, 2007, that I needed to begin dialysis as soon as possible. For the last 10 years, I have worked in sales, selling electrical components and data processing equipment like fiber-optic cable to contractors. When I learned I was starting dialysis, I met with my two bosses. I had already talked to them about my kidney problems, and they already had an idea that I would need to have dialysis treatments. They explained the benefits that were available and that I was covered for disability for 3 months. On June 5, 2007, I had a dialysis catheter inserted, and I began hemodialysis on June 6, 2007 at a dialysis center. I had another surgery to create an AV fistula in my left arm.

Being out of work was very hard. I felt weak and was depressed that I could not take care of my wife and daughter. Being home made me think too much. My wife was also depressed because she saw me being sad. Luckily, my one-year-old daughter did not understand what was going on. I enjoyed taking her out to the park because it took my mind off my problems.

Little by little, I felt stronger. I never thought I would miss my job, but I did. I was bored being home all day. After 3 months, I returned to work full time. At first, I had some of my accounts assigned to other people, but I soon was back to my old schedule. I tried to do some work while I was on hemodialysis, but the lack of an Internet connection was a problem. Sometimes after dialysis, I work at home until 1:00 a.m. I've had a lot of energy since starting dialysis and enjoy being back at work. I never complain about my job anymore.

27. Am I too old to receive dialysis treatments?

No! You are not too old to consider dialysis treatments at any age. Patients in their late 90s have been treated with dialysis. The most important requirement for patients considering dialysis at any age is a positive mental attitude and the desire to get better.

In the early days of dialysis treatments, the 1970s, older patients were not considered good candidates for dialysis treatments. The hemodialysis machines were primitive compared to today's equipment. Peritoneal dialysis was not readily available for continuous treatments on an outpatient basis. The availability of dialysis was limited to a few centers. Elderly patients were often treated conservatively, and not even offered dialysis as an option.

A great deal has changed. The modern hemodialysis machine allows older and sicker patients to receive treatments. The dialysate used for dialysis in the 1970s contained a substance called acetate. This acetate could pass through the dialysis membrane into the patient's blood. The acetate was then converted to **bicarbonate** to treat the accumulation of acids in the body. In the 1980s, technology changed to allow bicarbonate to be added directly to the dialysate, resulting in gentler and smoother treatments. It reduced the number of times the patient's blood pressure would fall during the treatment. More fluid could be removed safely. Patients with heart conditions could be treated without developing chest pain or other cardiac symptoms. Infirm and weak patients were able to tolerate hemodialysis.

The computer revolution has also improved the modern hemodialysis machine. Microprocessors are part of every machine. These small computers accurately measure how fast and how much fluid is removed. Microprocessors measure the composition and temperature of the dialysate. They detect leaking of blood through the dialysate membrane into the dialysate. Peritoneal dialysis has also benefited by modern technological advances.

The modern hemodialysis machine allows older and sicker patients to receive treatments.

Dialysis

Bicarbonate

A salt of carbonic acid that acts as an important buffer to help keep our blood from becoming too acidic.

Better tubing and connection systems have decreased the rate of infection. Peritoneal dialysis machines or cyclers that automatically perform dialysis benefited from microprocessors. Computers have made dialysis better and safer.

The improvement in medical care has helped older patients receive dialysis treatments. Better cardiac care including coronary artery bypass surgery, coronary angioplasty and stent placement, and implantable defibrillators have improved the life expectancy and quality of elderly patients' lives. Medications have also improved outcomes. The treatment of elevated blood pressure and cholesterol has contributed to people living longer.

In 2003, 26% of new patients beginning dialysis were older than 75 years of age. It is now common for patients over 90 years of age to begin dialysis treatments. Elderly patients are often afraid of dialysis treatments. They feel that treatments may be painful. A common fear is that once you start dialysis you will be trapped on dialysis and will not be able to stop treatment. Both of these fears are best addressed by talking to other elderly patients who are receiving dialysis treatments. Your healthcare professional can arrange for you to tour a dialysis center and to talk to patients while they are actually on dialysis. Most dialysis patients are happy to share their stories and have unique insight into dialysis treatments. They remember vividly what beginning dialysis was like and will honestly answer your questions.

Often the worst part of beginning dialysis is our fear of the unknown. It is impossible to predict who will do well on dialysis and who will not. Many elderly patients surprise themselves and the healthcare team. They expect to survive a few months. After a year or two on dialysis, they have gained strength, are more active, and are glad to have begun dialysis. If you do not know if dialysis is for you, you can give it a try for several months. You can always stop treatment.

28. Can I catch HIV or hepatitis from my dialysis treatment?

There has never been a case of a person contracting HIV (human immunodeficiency virus) from dialysis treatments. HIV can be transmitted by blood transfusions, needle sticks, sexual activity, and by sharing needles while using drugs. It cannot be transmitted by casual contact such as shaking hands, kissing, sitting in the same chair, or using the same toilet as an HIV-infected person. Accurate tests have been developed for HIV allowing the screening of blood donors and making our blood supply safe. It is necessary to get a person's permission to test them for HIV. Some states have laws restricting access to information concerning HIV in the medical record. Orally administered medicines now exist that can greatly reduce the amount of virus in an HIV-infected individual's body. This medical advance has allowed HIV patients to live a more normal life and has greatly improved their longevity.

In hemodialysis, all the tubing that comes into contact with blood is discarded after use. Some centers will reuse the dialysis membrane many times. The membrane is disinfected, carefully tested, and used only on the same person. There is no risk of getting HIV infection or hepatitis from reusing dialysis membranes. Unfortunately, needle sticks can occur in hemodialysis units. They usually involve staff members sticking themselves with a used needle from a patient. This may put the staff member at risk but does not pose a threat to the patient. Some hemodialysis centers allow patients to receive blood transfusions for anemia while they are on hemodialysis. The use of a medication called erythropoietin as well as the use of intravenous iron replacement has decreased the need for transfusions in dialysis patients. Because of the screening of blood donors, the blood supply in the United States and most countries is very safe. The chance of contracting HIV infection or hepatitis from blood transfusion is very small.

In the 1970s there were epidemics of hepatitis B infection in hemodialysis centers. This risk was recognized, and it was decided to treat patients with hepatitis B in special isolation areas within the dialysis unit, dramatically decreasing the transmission of hepatitis B. Today, all dialysis patients and dialysis staff are offered vaccination for hepatitis B. This series of three shots is your best defense against hepatitis B, and I urge you to take the hepatitis B vaccine.

More patients on dialysis have been exposed to hepatitis C infection than to hepatitis B. Hepatitis C is transmitted by blood transfusions, needle sticks, or sharing needles during intravenous drug use. Hepatitis C is not thought to be transmitted by sexual activity. Dialysis is not a risk factor for the transmission of hepatitis C. Most cases are asymptomatic, and people find out that they have been exposed to hepatitis C when blood tests are taken. Most people with hepatitis C recover. A small number of people develop chronic hepatitis, which if left untreated can result in permanent scarring or cirrhosis of the liver. Treatment is available to prevent this scarring, and it is important to have a thorough evaluation if you have chronic hepatitis C to see if you can benefit from treatment. There is no vaccine for hepatitis C. There is a third type of hepatitis called hepatitis A, which can be transmitted by eating contaminated food. People usually recover with no chronic scarring of the liver. A vaccine is available and should be taken when you travel to areas with a high risk of infection, or if you suffer from chronic hepatitis B or C infection to prevent further damage to your liver. Hepatitis A is rare in dialysis patients in the United States.

Home dialysis patients must take special precautions to protect family and household members from exposure to blood, dialysate, and used dialysis needles. These precautions are called **universal precautions** because they are always used all the time with everyone. They involve washing hands before and after contact with a patient. Family members should also wear eye shields, gloves, and protective gowns when close enough to the dialysis procedure to be at risk for blood splashing on them. It does not matter if your family member on dialysis is HIV negative or does not have hepatitis. We still use universal precautions. This is because there are patients who are in what we call the window period of infection, which refers to the early stages of HIV or hepatitis infection. The patient is exposed to the disease, and viruses are reproducing in their body. Their body has not yet made antibodies to the virus. The test for HIV or hepatitis is negative, but the person can still be contagious. The other reason for universal precautions is that some family members may find it difficult to reveal to their loved ones that they have an infection.

Universal precautions

Wearing medical gloves, goggles, and face shields to avoid contact with body fluids such as blood and peritoneal fluid. Universal precautions protect us from the risk of transmission of blood-borne diseases such as hepatitis and HIV-AIDS.

Dialysis

Universal precautions are like looking both ways before crossing the street. If you learn good habits in the beginning, you will be able to avoid an accident for many years to come. If you are splashed with blood from a family member, the first thing to do is wash the blood off. If the splash has gotten into your eye, irrigating the eye with tap water should be done immediately. If you stick yourself with a used needle, again immediately wash the needle stick site with soap and water. Report the needle stick to your doctor or to your family member's doctor. They can counsel you and your family member to determine if special tests for HIV or hepatitis are needed. Most people splashed with blood or dialysate, or who experience a needle stick have nothing serious happen to them.

PART THREE

Preparing to Begin Dialysis

What is a nephrologist?

How does my doctor know I need dialysis?

What is a shunt or access for dialysis?

More ...

29. What is a nephrologist?

A nephrologist is a medical doctor who has received specialized training in the diagnosis and treatment of kidney diseases. After 4 years of college and 4 years of medical school, an MD or DO (Doctor of Osteopathy) degree is awarded. The nephrologist has also received 3 years of training as a resident in internal medicine where he or she has studied and managed a large number of different medical problems. After completing the residency in internal medicine, the nephrologist will have 2 or more years of fellowship training in nephrology. The fellow will work under the supervision of several experienced nephrologists who are board certified by the American Board of Internal Medicine. These teachers have years of experience in diagnosing and treating patients with kidney disorders. Many of them have conducted research and have written papers on renal disease. Under their guidance, the fellow will learn to diagnose and a large number of kidney diseases.

The training will include working in a hospital and taking care of critically ill patients in the intensive care unit and the emergency department. The fellow will also learn about hemodialysis and peritoneal dialysis, both in the hospital and in the dialysis center. Kidney biopsy and kidney pathology are studied. The fellow will learn about renal transplantation as an option for treating kidney failure. Many fellowship programs require that the fellow be involved in research. The high point of the fellow's training could be presenting his or her research at a national kidney meeting such as the annual meeting of the **American Society of Nephrology**. This national meeting attracts up to 15,000 nephrologists to hear talks and papers pre-

American Society of Nephrology

A national organization of physicians and scientists founded in 1966 to study and treat kidney disease.

sented from the best nephrologists from all over the world. In addition, fellows will attend many conferences at their hospital. Some fellows will take a third year to specialize in transplant medicine, critical care medicine, or other subspecialties of nephrology. They may take an extra year of research. After their fellowship training, fellows can take an examination for board certification by the American Board of Internal Medicine.

The idea of having a floor of the hospital dedicated to the study, teaching, and treatment of kidney disease was first established by Richard Bright (1789–1858) at the Guy's Hospital and Medical School in London, England. His association of the finding of protein in the urine and the diagnosis of kidney disease is still important today. In his honor, the condition of having protein in the urine was called Bright's disease. Many physicians after Dr. Bright were interested in kidney disease, but the modern era of nephrology began in the 1940s. Physicians studying the physiology (or the way the kidney works) began to make great progress. Experimental dialysis treatment was begun in the 1940s and 1950s. In 1954, the first kidney transplant was performed. Physicians developed a method of performing kidney biopsies without surgery by inserting a needle through the skin and obtaining a small piece of tissue to examine under the microscope. In 1960, an association called the International Society of Nephrology held its first meeting in Evian, France. The American Society of Nephrology was founded in 1966. All these advances promoted the establishment of nephrology as an active subspecialty of internal medicine. The development of formal training in nephrology has allowed patients with kidney disease to receive the latest treatment available.

The development of formal training in nephrology has allowed patients with kidney disease to receive the latest treatment available.

If your doctor has diagnosed a kidney problem or if you have a family history of a genetic kidney disease, it is advisable to ask your doctor or healthcare professional for a referral to see a nephrologist. The nephrologist will concentrate on diagnosing the cause of the kidney problem and will attempt to cure or stabilize the problem. The earlier the evaluation, the more likely it will be that the problem can be reversed or stabilized. The hope of early intervention is to prevent or delay the need for kidney dialysis.

30. What is a urologist?

A **urologist** is a medical doctor who specializes in the treatment of diseases of the kidney and urinary tract. Like a nephrologist, the urologist has spent 4 years attending medical school. After graduation, the urologist will spend 1 year training in general surgery followed by 4 or 5 years of residency training in urology. The urologist, as a surgeon, will concentrate on problems such as diseases of the prostate, kidney tumors, kidney stones, and disorders of the bladder. He or she will learn **cystoscopy**, a procedure in which a small fiber-optic tube is inserted in the bladder. Disorders of the bladder and urinary tract can be diagnosed and treated without making a cut or surgical incision. Tubes called **stents** can be inserted during cystoscopy to bypass a blockage caused by a stone or tumor and allow the kidneys to function. A urologist may become skilled in **laparoscopic surgery**, which allows surgery to be done through small incisions in the abdomen, allowing a faster recovery time. After completing the residency training program, urologists can become board certified by the American Board of Urology. They will have to give case presentations of patients

Urologist

A physician who specializes in the diagnosis and treatment of diseases of the kidney and urinary tract. Urologists have training in surgical procedures used in the treatment of prostate problems, tumors of the urinary tract, and the removal of kidney stones.

Cystoscopy

A surgical procedure performed by a urologist in which a small fiber-optic tube called a cystoscope is inserted through the urethra into the bladder. The urologist can diagnose tumors of the bladder and can perform biopsies and other procedures through the cystoscope.

Stent

A medical device that looks like a hollow tube. Stents are inserted across blocked blood arteries to the heart, kidneys, and other organs to increase the blood flow. Other kinds of stents are also used to treat blockages in the ureters that transport urine from the kidneys to the bladder.

they have cared for and pass three examinations to prove competency in urology.

Urologists were important in the development of peritoneal and hemodialysis. A urologist, Dr. J. Hartwell Harrison, was a member of the team that performed the first renal transplant from one identical twin to another at the Peter Bent Brigham Hospital in Boston, Massachusetts, in 1954. As the specialty of nephrology developed, urologists spent less time with dialysis and renal failure and concentrated more on surgical diseases of the kidney. However, nephrologists and urologists have continued to work together on many diseases. Patients suffering from kidney stones will have them removed by urologists. The nephrologist will help treat the patient to prevent more stones from forming. Many times patients are not sure if they should see a urologist or nephrologist as a kidney specialist. You can ask your primary care doctor which is the appropriate kidney doctor for you. Often the urologist will determine that you should see a nephrologist if medical kidney disease is suspected.

Laparoscopic surgery
Surgery performed under general anesthesia by inserting fiber-optic tubes through several small incisions.

Preparing to Begin Dialysis

31. How does my doctor know I need dialysis?

The evaluation to determine if a person needs dialysis begins with the medical history. Your doctor will ask you questions regarding your health in the past. He or she will ask about symptoms of kidney failure. Early symptoms of kidney failure include a decreased appetite, weight loss, hiccups, nausea or vomiting, and a bitter or metallic taste in your mouth. A general physical examination will be performed. The doctor will measure your blood pressure, examine your heart,

Early symptoms of kidney failure include a decreased appetite, weight loss, hiccups, nausea or vomiting, and a bitter or metallic taste in your mouth.

Anemia

A decrease in the number of red blood cells present in the blood, which can be due to blood loss or a decreased production of red blood cells due to iron deficiency, poor nutrition, or disease. Decreased red blood cell survival occurs in kidney disease. Symptoms of anemia include fatigue, weakness, and shortness of breath on exertion.

lungs, and abdomen, and look for evidence of fluid retention in your legs and feet, and around your eyes. Blood and urine tests will be ordered.

One of the most important blood tests is the BUN test, or blood urea nitrogen test. This was the first blood test developed to measure kidney function. As a person's renal function gets worse, the kidney's ability to excrete or remove urea from the blood declines. The urea level in the blood increases. Another important blood test is the creatinine level. Creatinine is a substance produced from our muscles. As the creatinine enters the bloodstream, it is filtered and excreted by the kidneys. As kidney function decreases, the level of creatinine in the blood increases because less creatinine is removed. Another important blood test is for potassium level. If the potassium level is too high, the patient may be at risk for heart problems. A hematocrit and hemoglobin test can determine if you have an **anemia** or low red blood cell count. Anemia is a common finding in kidney failure. A sonogram can be helpful to evaluate the size of the kidneys. Small kidney size can indicate that the kidneys are scarred and are less likely to improve. A 24-hour collection of urine for creatinine clearance can measure the amount of kidney function a person has left and is more accurate than blood tests. This test is done at home and will require you to save all the urine you make during a 24-hour period. If you get up at night to urinate, you must remember to save this urine. After collecting the urine, you will go to the lab or doctor's office to obtain a blood creatinine level to calculate your kidney function.

In some patients, the decision to start dialysis is easy. They look and feel sick. Fluid is building up in their body, and they are short of breath. They have nausea, vomiting, and cannot eat. In these patients, emergency dialysis can be life saving. They often feel much better after one or two dialysis treatments. This makes accepting the need for dialysis treatments much easier. In other patients, these dramatic symptoms are not present. If toxins and poisons from kidney failure build up gradually, the person will adapt and be able to tolerate the kidney failure. This can make the decision to start dialysis more difficult because the person feels well. Despite blood tests showing kidney failure, the symptoms of kidney failure are absent.

In the early days of dialysis, because resources were limited, almost all patients became ill with symptoms. We have learned that it is better not to wait until the last possible moment before starting dialysis. Early intervention helps prevent damage to the heart, nerves, and bones. Doctors often cannot precisely predict when these organs will be damaged. In general, when the creatinine clearance is 18 to 20 mL/minute we begin preparing the patient for dialysis, and we begin dialysis when the creatinine clearance is 12 to 15 mL/minute. This is to keep the patient out of danger. We have learned after years of experience that it is better to start dialysis before a crisis occurs. The first treatment can be scheduled at a specific time, and family members can be available to support the patient psychologically. When starting dialysis is delayed, individuals might have to start dialysis on an emergency basis, requiring them to go to an emergency room during the middle of the night or on a weekend. Their regular doctor might not be available to help treat them.

Because many patients adapt to kidney failure, they often tell me after starting dialysis that they did not realize how bad they actually had felt. Their appetite improves and they regain their taste for their favorite food. They are stronger and can walk faster and longer before getting tired. High blood pressure is often easier to control after starting dialysis because fluid is removed efficiently. Some patients can decrease their blood pressure medications after starting dialysis. Their sense of well-being improves. They no longer have to worry if they will get sick or have an emergency and need to be rushed to the hospital for emergency dialysis.

32. How will my doctor help me prepare for dialysis?

In the most optimal situation, you will meet your doctor before you need to begin dialysis. He or she will discuss dialysis with you and your family and will have reviewed your blood and other tests. The most important thing that your doctor can do at this stage is give you information. The more you understand dialysis, the less frightening it will be. When I began my career in nephrology, we would carefully explain the dialysis procedure to patients and answer their many questions. Now, many doctors will also mention every possible bad outcome even if the chance of that bad outcome is very unlikely. It is important to tell your doctor how much information you feel comfortable receiving. Some patients need to hear about every detail. Others will put themselves in the hands of someone they trust and let them make many of the decisions. Too much information can sometimes be overwhelming. Many patients want a family member or friend to come with them and receive a lot of the information. That person can be your advocate and help you ask questions and make decisions. Some patients learn that they will need dialysis as an emergency and need to begin dialysis right away. Although this news can be very stressful, dialysis is a very safe and effective procedure and the overwhelming majority of patients tolerate their dialysis treatment without difficulty.

Your doctor will discuss the need to create an access for your dialysis treatment. In hemodialysis, the best access is called an a-v fistula (**Figure 4**). This small tube in the arm is created by connecting an artery to a vein during a surgical procedure under local anesthesia. The fistula may take several months to mature due to the thickening of the wall of the vein of the fistula's vein or because of an increased pressure from the arterial blood. When the fistula is mature or ready for use, needles are inserted into the fistula to obtain the blood for the dialysis treatment. The early creation of the a-v fistula can make beginning dialysis easier and safer. A peritoneal dialysis access or catheter takes less time to be ready than an a-v fistula. Most catheters are ready to use in about 2 weeks.

Part of the care you will receive before beginning dialysis is learning the diet you need to follow to keep yourself healthy. In many instances, this diet will include a restriction in the amount of sodium and potassium you will be able to eat. Phosphorus found in meat and dairy products may be restricted. Phosphate binders, medicines that are taken with food, can also decrease the phosphorus that is absorbed by the gastrointestinal tract. Many patients mistakenly believe that drinking extra fluid will be helpful in kidney disease. This is often wrong. Drink if you are thirsty, but avoid drinking extra fluid. The best person to counsel

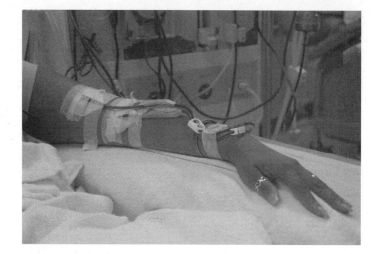

Figure 4　A-V fistula
Source: K. Neelakantappa, MD

you on your diet is a dietitian who has experience with dialysis patients.

Many patients with kidney failure begin to develop anemia as part of their renal failure because the survival of the red blood cells is decreased. Erythropoietin, a hormone produced by the kidney, is decreased in kidney failure. Erythropoietin is a messenger that tells our bone marrow to increase the production of red blood cells. The erythropoietin and other medications with similar action can be given by subcutaneous injection to increase the production of red blood cells. This injection can be given every week and will decrease the symptoms of anemia that can include weakness, shortness of breath, and pale skin. Many patients also have to take iron supplements with the erythropoietin injection to increase their red blood cell production.

Due to an inability to eliminate or excrete phosphorus from the body, patients with kidney failure often begin to have bone problems before they need dialysis treatments. This increase in phosphorus in the bloodstream causes calcium, the major element in bones, to be deposited back into the bones. This low calcium can stimulate **parathyroid hormone (PTH)** production. Parathyroid hormone is produced by four small glands in the neck that are near the thyroid gland. Overactive parathyroid glands can produce too much parathyroid hormone, which can cause re-absorption of bone and can lead to aches, pains, and in extreme cases bone fractures. Another symptom of too much parathyroid hormone is itching.

Your doctor will continue to focus on control of your blood pressure and blood sugar if you are a diabetic. Many patients with kidney failure have an elevated cholesterol level as well as elevated triglycerides. This condition is controlled with diet, exercise, and sometimes medication.

By now, you are thinking that preparing for dialysis is a lot of work and not much fun. Many patients find all these problems overwhelming and depressing. Every situation is different. Many patients have no symptoms of anemia, bone disease and make enough urine to not require a very restrictive diet. These individual differences are why you need to communicate well with your doctor and concentrate on the most important aspects of your care.

Parathyroid hormone (PTH)

A hormone made and released by the chief cells of the four parathyroid glands found in the neck to regulate calcium metabolism.

Due to an inability to eliminate or excrete phosphorus from the body, patients with kidney failure often begin to have bone problems before they need dialysis treatments.

33. Will I need to be hospitalized to begin my dialysis treatments?

Many patients who have time to prepare for their dialysis treatments will not have to be hospitalized overnight. If your medical condition is stable, and you have a good support system at home, you may begin dialysis as an outpatient. Most of the time, the dialysis access can be created as an outpatient procedure. If your access is in place and ready to use, you can start hemodialysis as an outpatient. Patients beginning peritoneal dialysis will come to the dialysis unit several days a week for training. They may be receiving hemodialysis treatments three times a week during the training until they feel competent in performing their own peritoneal dialysis.

Different dialysis units have different levels of care. Dialysis units in hospitals sometimes have a mixture of inpatients and outpatients. These units have a high nurse to patient ratio. Physicians spend more time in the unit because the patients on dialysis require a higher level of care. The hospital units have beds as well as dialysis chairs because they take care of weaker and more debilitated patients. When patients become stronger and more stable on dialysis, they can be transferred to an outpatient unit that is closer to home. If your medical condition is unstable, or if you have a heart problem, have had recent major surgery, bleeding, or a stroke, you may have to start dialysis as an inpatient. Many patients feel safe and secure in the hospital. As their condition improves, they can continue their treatment as an outpatient.

A great number of patients still meet their nephrologist for the first time when they need urgent or emergency dialysis. This may be because they have not been referred to a nephrologist by their primary care doctor, or they may have been reluctant to see the nephrologist because of fears of starting dialysis. Many people in the United States and other countries do not receive preventative general medical visits. This decreases their chance of receiving treatment that may keep them off dialysis. In general, the sooner you are evaluated the better.

34. I feel that I would rather die than go on dialysis. Is this a common feeling?

Many patients when confronted with beginning dialysis feel that their life is over. I once went to a national conference on dialysis attended by kidney doctors and dialysis nurses where we were asked to choose our own therapy if we were to develop kidney failure. The choices were hemodialysis, peritoneal dialysis, or no dialysis. To my surprise, a significant number of these healthcare workers, about 6%, stated that they would choose not to go on dialysis and to die. These feelings of helplessness have nothing to do with educational level or knowledge about dialysis. Patients with other diseases such as heart disease, diabetes, or cancer have similar feelings. They are a normal part of coping with illness and are part of the recovery process. Having a medical problem changes our idea of who we are. We feel vulnerable, inadequate, and imperfect. These feelings are signs of **depression** that all dialysis patients experience. They decrease with time. Talking about refusing dialysis is often very upsetting to the patient, the patient's family, and sometimes to the medical staff. I find that expressing these emotions rather than suppressing them is important and helpful in the

Depression

A medical term used to describe feelings of intense sadness, loss of interest in activities of daily life, and a decreased appetite and sense of well-being.

healing process. All dialysis patients will have these feelings, some often, others infrequently. The best response is to listen to why the patient feels this way and to avoid stating that these feelings are uncalled for or abnormal. Some patients will voice their concerns to family members but not the dialysis team. At our outpatient dialysis unit, we have a **psychologist** who is available to talk to all patients about this and other issues.

The overwhelming number of patients needing dialysis accept treatment, and most do very well. Although the number is very small, some patients choose to not begin dialysis or decide to stop dialysis when their condition deteriorates and their quality of life is very poor. These patients are often elderly and have multiple medical problems. Art Buchwald, the noted columnist and Pulitzer Prize winner, developed acute renal failure in his 80s. He tried dialysis but decided it was not for him and stopped. His kidneys recovered enough for him to survive for a period of time. He wrote a book called *Too Soon to Say Goodbye*, in which he discusses his serious medical problems. He faces medical illness the same way he faced the rest of his life, with humor and good spirits. Most people relate to illness the same way they relate to their life when they are well, even more so. Chronic procrastinators will find a million excuses to delay beginning dialysis until the last minute. Depressed people will become more depressed. People who are decisive and organized in their daily lives will get all the information they can, research which doctor is best for them, and take action to remain healthy.

It is important to realize that the decision to start dialysis is not irrevocable. I often tell my patients who are

---

Psychologist

A healthcare professional who works with patients on their mental health problems including depression and anxiety.

The overwhelming number of patients needing dialysis accept treatment, and most do very well.

reluctant to begin dialysis to try one dialysis treatment. This makes them understand that they are in control of their treatment. After their first treatment, they realize that dialysis is not that bad and it is something that will help them lead a better and more productive life. Patients may be candidates for a kidney transplant in the future, which will enable them to get off dialysis. Accepting dialysis is 90% of the struggle. The adjustment period to dialysis is about 6 months. At 6 months, if you are still depressed and find dialysis extremely difficult, you may want to see a psychologist or psychiatrist. Medications for depression work well in patients on dialysis and may be helpful to patients who are severely depressed.

Erick Lucero writes:

Before I knew I needed dialysis, I used to take my uncle home from his dialysis treatments. He is older than I am and was often weak after his dialysis treatments. When my nephrologist told me that I would need dialysis, I knew that dialysis would take a lot of time and effort, and would interfere with my life. I had a sad feeling and was scared. Before beginning dialysis, I was very tired. I went to sleep after coming home from work. I started dialysis after my nephrologist found that my blood tests had gotten worse. My wife speaks of that day as "the black day," as if she was in mourning. After beginning dialysis, I began to feel better. I was less tired and had more energy. I spent time with my young daughter who helped take my mind off my problems. After 3 months, I returned to work. I was bored not working and felt better after beginning hemodialysis. Being on dialysis is less stressful than waiting to begin dialysis. When you are on dialysis, you know what to expect. You fall into a routine. When I am on hemodialysis, I am taking care of my health. The rest of the time, I am involved with my family, my friends, and work. Since I feel better on dialysis, I am less sad.

35. What is a shunt or access for dialysis?

Shunt

An old term used to describe an access used to obtain blood for hemodialysis. It initially referred to the Quinton-Scribner shunt first used in the 1960s. Today, the term includes the a-v fistula and a-v graft which "shunt" blood from the artery to the vein, bypassing the small capillaries.

A **shunt** is an old term that has survived from the early days of hemodialysis. It was first used to describe a device invented by Dr. Belding Scribner and Dr. Wayne Quinton to obtain blood for hemodialysis treatments. In the early days of dialysis, a tube or catheter was placed in an artery by a surgical procedure. Blood was removed from the artery and would run through plastic tubing to the hemodialysis machine. Blood would then run back to the patient into another tube that was placed in a vein. Each artery and vein could only be used once. This limited the number of dialysis treatments because patients ran out of usable arteries and veins. Drs. Scribner and Quinton began working on a device that could be used for many dialysis treatments. They inserted Teflon-coated tubing into an artery and a vein in the patient's arms. After dialysis was completed, the two plastic tubes, one in an artery and one in a vein, were connected together. The tubing was outside the skin, and blood flowing through the tubing on a continuous basis prevented clotting. This shunt, which allowed blood to flow from an artery to a vein, bypassing small blood vessels, was first used in 1960. It was later improved by using flexible silicon plastic tubing. This Quinton-Scribner shunt revolutionized hemodialysis and allowed many patients to be treated with hemodialysis for temporary or acute kidney failure. Dr. Scribner's shunt enabled him to treat patients for months and then years. He organized the first dialysis unit for chronic patients who could not recover kidney function at the University of Washington Hospital. In time, even though the Quinton-Scribner shunt is no longer used, the word shunt became used to describe any device that enabled blood to flow from an artery to a vein that is used for hemodialysis. The term dialysis access is a more modern term for shunt. It means a device that allows access to obtain blood from the circulation to perform dialysis.

The best type of access for hemodialysis is an **arterial-venous fistula**, or a-v fistula for short. Instead of using plastic tubing to connect an artery to a vein, the artery is directly connected to the vein by a vascular surgeon. The a-v fistula is usually located in the arm. The operation, done under local anesthesia, causes blood from the artery to go directly into the vein without passing through small blood vessels called capillaries. Blood is "shunted" from an artery to a vein. This arterial blood is under a higher pressure because it is pumped by the heart. This high pressure causes the vein to dilate (become larger). The wall of the vein becomes thicker. After weeks to months, this dilated vein can be used for hemodialysis. This process is called maturation of the fistula. Two needles can be inserted through the skin into the a-v fistula. One needle carries blood out of the fistula to the dialysis machine. After the blood is cleaned of poisons and toxins, it is carried back to the fistula and is returned to the body by the second needle. Blood can be removed and returned continuously during the dialysis treatment. After dialysis is completed, the needles are removed from the fistula. The patient places a sterile gauze over the hole in the fistula until the a small blood clot seals the needle hole. A Band-Aid is then applied over the needle hole. The

Arterial-venous fistula

A tube that connects an artery to a vein and is constructed by a vascular surgeon. When mature, the a-v fistula can have needles inserted into it to carry blood through plastic tubing to and from the hemodialysis machine.

a-v fistula is the best access for dialysis because it is made of natural materials, artery, and vein. The fistula is capable of healing if damaged and is less likely to become infected. It can last a long time. I have many patients whose fistulas are still working after 20 or more years.

An **arterial-venous graft**, or a-v graft, is another type of access or shunt used in hemodialysis. The a-v graft is used in patients who cannot have an a-v fistula because their veins are small. Tubing made of a material called Gortex is connected between an artery and a vein by a vascular surgeon during an operation under local anesthesia. The tubing runs under the skin. Needles are inserted into the plastic tube to obtain blood for hemodialysis. Because the a-v graft is made of plastic, it cannot repair itself if damaged. It is more likely to become infected. If infected, it must be removed by a surgeon. On average, a-v grafts last 9 months to 2 or 3 years. They are not a good choice for patients who plan to spend many years on hemodialysis because they will need to be replaced many times.

Patients who do not have a permanent access who need dialysis can use a **catheter**. A catheter is a long plastic tube that is inserted into a vein. Local anesthesia, usually an injection of lidocaine, is used to numb the area. The catheter is sometimes inserted in a vein in the groin called the femoral vein. This procedure is done in the hospital or as an outpatient when dialysis needs to be done on a temporary basis. The catheter can be removed after the dialysis is completed, making it less likely for the catheter to become infected. Catheters can also be inserted in veins in the neck. They can be left in place for a period of time. Longer catheters are placed to come out of the skin in the

Arterial-venous graft

A length of gortex tubing connected between an artery and a vein that is created by a vascular surgeon. The a-v graft is tunneled under the skin to allow needles to be inserted into it to carry blood through plastic tubing to the hemodialysis machine.

Catheter

A plastic tube used for dialysis. Catheters are inserted into blood vessels to obtain blood for hemodialysis treatments. Peritoneal dialysis catheters are inserted in the abdomen, and are used to instill and drain dialysate into and out of the abdomen during peritoneal dialysis treatments.

upper chest. This positioning makes them less visible, as they are under the patient's shirt. Catheters can be used for hemodialysis immediately. There is no need to wait for the a-v fistula to develop or mature, for the surgical incisions to heal, or for swelling after surgery to decrease. The big disadvantage to catheters is a high chance of infection. The catheter comes out of the skin and is covered by a sterile dressing. Bacteria normally found on the skin can enter the opening in the skin and infect the catheter. Patients with catheters cannot take a bath or shower because this will get the catheter wet and increase the chance of infection. If the catheter becomes infected, antibiotics can be given and the catheter will need to be removed.

36. Should I begin dialysis before I really need it?

Most patients will try to delay dialysis as long as possible. This is a natural reaction. If kidney failure develops slowly, patients are able to adapt to the poisons and toxins in their blood. They may eat less protein, have a decreased appetite, and develop itching, hiccups, nausea, and vomiting. All of these symptoms can be tolerated if they are mild. Your remaining kidney function can be measured by a test called a 24-hour urine collection for creatinine clearance. A normal test result is 100 to 125 mL/minute. When the creatinine clearance decreases to 15 to 12 mL/min, it is time to begin dialysis. If you are a diabetic or elderly, you need to start dialysis a little earlier. You will not tolerate high levels of toxins and poisons in your blood as well as other patients. Fluid could also build up in your body and put a strain on your heart. If your appetite is poor, you may lose weight. Especially important is avoiding loss of muscle mass. When we do not eat enough calories, our bodies use fat stores and break down muscle for food. This can result in you being increasingly weak and less able to perform your daily activities. Carrying groceries, getting to work, cleaning your home can all become increasingly difficult if you lose muscle mass and body weight. It is important to look for this loss of weight. Because most patients do not want to begin dialysis, they can easily rationalize that they are fine. They can minimize the symptoms of renal failure, but weight loss is objective evidence that it would be better to begin dialysis.

Neuropathy

Damage to the peripheral nerves of the body. Symptoms include tingling in the hands and feet, weakness, and numbness.

Patients with kidney failure can also develop nerve damage, or **neuropathy**. This begins as numbness in the toes, feet, and hands. This neuropathy is progressive and can lead to weakness of the arms and legs. It can be treated with dialysis. Anemia, or low red blood cell count, is another problem that improves with dialysis. Anemia can cause weakness, fatigue, shortness of breath, and chest pain. An elevated potassium level, swelling in the legs, abdomen, or around the eyes, and an increased amount of acid in the blood are all signs that you need to start dialysis.

In the 1970s when dialysis was not readily available and there was a lack of knowledge about dialysis among patients and doctors, it was common to have patients at death's door before they were started on dialysis. We have learned that doctors are not that skilled in predicting exactly when you must begin dialysis. You may feel fine one day, and be seriously ill the next. It is always better to begin dialysis in a calm and predictable manner. It is terrible to become ill in the middle of the night, be rushed to an emergency room where the doctors and nurses are not familiar with your case, and begin dialysis on an emergency basis. For all these reasons, it is better to begin dialysis before you think you really need it. You may end up on dialysis a few weeks earlier, but you will preserve your strength and sense of well-being. You will decrease the stress and anxiety of your family. Often the worst part of beginning dialysis is thinking about it. Once you commit to starting dialysis, you will have less fear of the future and the unknown. This will make your adjustment to dialysis so much easier and allow you to continue to do the things you want in life.

You may feel fine one day, and be seriously ill the next.

37. Who will help me find out if my insurance covers my dialysis treatments?

Dialysis treatments are expensive, about $30,000 to $50,000 a year. Most medical insurance will cover all or most of the cost of dialysis treatments as a life-saving medical treatment. If you know that you will need dialysis in the future, you should try to meet with a social worker who has experience working with dialysis patients. Every dialysis unit has a social worker who has experience in counseling patients about health insurance. They will be able to help you understand what your insurance does and does not cover. Medicare covers 80% of the costs of dialysis, and patients will need to have a supplementary insurance policy that covers the remaining 20%. Some insurance plans do not cover the cost of medications taken at home. The average dialysis patient takes 8 to 12 medications a day. It is important to try to obtain a prescription plan that will cover the costs of these medications. Medicare has established a plan called part D in 2007, which pays the cost of medications for some patients. Drug companies have programs available for patients who cannot afford their medications and who do not qualify for other programs. The National Kidney Foundation also has grants that can help pay for medications on a one time basis.

Approximately 45 million Americans have no health insurance coverage at all. Uninsured patients who need dialysis are not uncommon. Fortunately, in the United States, no one is denied dialysis treatments because of an inability to pay. The federal government has provided insurance through the Medicaid and Medicare programs. If you have worked and paid taxes, you will be eligible for Medicare coverage 3 months after your first dialysis treatment. Medicaid eligibility will vary from state to state and is income based. It is important to discuss your eligibility with the dialysis or hospital social worker or have your relatives or significant other help you with the application process. Patients who are from other countries legally or illegally are eligible for Medicaid, which pays for emergency dialysis only. Emergency Medicaid for dialysis will not pay for medications, transportation, or doctors visits. The cost of transportation to and from the dialysis center can be significant, especially if the dialysis center is far from home.

Home dialysis patients have their own financial issues. The transportation costs to and from the dialysis center are much less. After their training is complete, they can expect to go to the dialysis center once a month if their condition is stable. Home hemodialysis patients have several additional expenses. The dialysis machine, dialyzers, tubing needles, gauze, and many other supplies are paid for by the insurance. The plumbing for the water for dialysis needs to be equipped with a backflow preventer. Waste lines to discard used dialysate may also need to be installed. The cost of the initial plumbing work could range from $1,000 to $2,000 and is not covered by insurance. The hemodialysis machine requires a dedicated electrical connection with 20 amperes of current. It will also need a ground fault circuit interrupter (GFCI) to turn off the electricity in the event of a short circuit. Your electricity and water bill will increase if you are on home hemodialysis. The cost of a recliner chair may not be covered by your insurance. The cost of home peritoneal dialysis is much less expensive than home hemodialysis. The main requirement for peritoneal dialysis is storage space for supplies.

Financial matters create a great deal of anxiety for patients and their families beginning dialysis. Many people are not used to discussing financial matters with their doctors. Kidney doctors usually have a great deal of experience dealing with patients with social and financial problems. They may not know the answer to your question, but they will know who on the healthcare team is best equipped to work on your problem with you.

38. Will dialysis heal my damaged kidneys?

Dialysis treatments are a renal replacement therapy. Dialysis replaces some of the functions that your kidneys provide. Dialysis does not heal your kidneys. Additional treatment will be required to heal your kidneys. The type of treatment will depend on the cause of your kidney disease. If you have a blockage to your

Glomerulonephritis

An inflammation of the filter or glomerulus of the kidney caused by many diseases.

Uremia

Symptoms caused by kidney failure that include loss of appetite, itching, hiccups, nausea, vomiting, seizures, and lethargy.

kidneys, surgery or the insertion of a tube or stent to bypass the blockage may be the treatment needed. If you have an inflammation of the kidneys called **glomerulonephritis**, you may be treated with immunosuppressive medications. Patients who have kidney failure due to medications will sometimes improve with time after the medicine has been stopped. The chance of your kidneys healing and of you getting off of dialysis depends on the amount of scarring of your kidneys that has occurred. Dialysis will keep you in good physical and nutritional shape while your doctors diagnose and treat your underlying kidney problem. Dialysis helps you by removing poisons and toxins, fluid, and electrolytes like potassium. It will remove acids that build up in the body. Dialysis can also remove certain medications and vitamins that are beneficial (see Question 25). Many patients have reported a decrease in the amount of urine they produce after starting dialysis. This is very common and does not mean that dialysis is making your kidneys worse. It is a common misconception that dialysis is responsible for some of the conditions associated with kidney failure such as neuropathy, anemia, or bone disease. It is actually the toxins and poisons that build up in the body that are responsible for these conditions, not the dialysis treatment. The buildup of toxins and poisons in the body is called **uremia**. Because dialysis cannot remove all the toxins and poisons, it is an imperfect treatment. Patients who receive more dialysis treatment time have less complications of kidney failure. The more you learn about dialysis by reading, talking to the dialysis team, and attending educational programs about renal failure, the better equipped you will be to actively participate in your care.

39. Can Jehovah's Witnesses be treated with dialysis?

Jehovah's Witnesses are members of a church that number one million people in the United States and six million people worldwide. Jehovah's Witnesses have a deeply held religious belief that they should not accept blood transfusions. They will not accept whole blood or parts of blood such as red blood cells, white blood cells, platelets, plasma, or serum albumin infusions. Jehovah's Witnesses are not against receiving medical care. I have taken care of many Jehovah's Witnesses, and all of them have accepted hemodialysis treatments. It is important to help minimize the possibility of blood loss to prevent the need for transfusion. This can be done by starting these patients on a medication called erythropoietin early in the course of their renal failure. Erythropoietin is a naturally occurring substance that is produced by the kidneys. It stimulates the production of red blood cells in the bone marrow. Erythropoietin is now manufactured and can be given by injection. Other brand names for erythropoietin are Epogen and Procrit.

Iron supplements given in pills or by intravenous injection can also be helpful. If the red blood cell level in the body is maintained at a near-normal level, the chance that a blood transfusion will be needed will be greatly reduced. It is also important to avoid blood thinners such as aspirin, Coumadin, Plavix, and other medications that can prevent the blood from clotting. If a surgical procedure is needed, a surgeon who is experienced in low-blood–loss surgery should be consulted. If bleeding occurs, a synthetically made product called recombinant factor VII is accepted by most Jehovah's Witnesses because it is not obtained from a blood donor. Kidney transplantation is not seen as the same as blood transfusions. Jehovah's Witnesses have received kidney, pancreas, liver, and bone marrow transplants. There has been a trend in medicine to use fewer blood transfusions in all patients because of the risks of transfusions. In 2001, the Society for the Advancement of Blood Management was formed by health professionals who are interested in reducing transfusions (*www.sabm.org*). Because of their religious beliefs, Jehovah's Witnesses have stimulated healthcare workers to develop new strategies to reduce bleeding and transfusions. Several blood substitutes are currently being evaluated in scientific clinical trials. These advances have benefited all patients, regardless of their religious beliefs.

40. Why do I need hemodialysis three times a week?

Our kidneys work 24 hours a day, 7 days a week. They work when we are sleeping, going to work, and eating meals, and they remove fluids, salts, toxins, and medications on a continuous basis. Hemodialysis removes these substances on an intermittent basis. Peritoneal dialysis is a chronic therapy and is more similar to our normal kidneys. In the early days of dialysis treatment, it was recognized by physicians that one or two hemodialysis treatments a week were not enough because patients had poor outcomes. Because of these observations, three times a week hemodialysis became the standard therapy. Insurance companies recognized three times a week hemodialysis.

Recently, there has been an interest in daily hemodialysis. This therapy is more similar to our normal kidney function and can be accomplished by being on home dialysis with treatments every day. Some patients choose to have dialysis at night. This is known as **nocturnal hemodialysis**. Patients on daily hemodialysis have lower blood pressures because fluid is removed every day. They are on less medication. Their phosphorus levels are lower and they have more energy. Of course, daily dialysis requires a huge commitment by the patient. Many people prefer to have dialysis three times a week because it allows them four days without dialysis treatments. Many patients ask if they will be better off on daily hemodialysis. I tell them to try it. Most patients on daily hemodialysis do not return to three times a week dialysis because they feel better. They are able to eat more varied foods and to increase their fluid intake.

No one therapy is right for everyone. I have seen patients go from home dialysis to in-center dialysis because of medical problems that required them to be under closer medical and nursing supervision. After their condition improved, they were able to return to home dialysis.

Nocturnal hemodialysis

Hemodialysis treatments done at night six or seven days a week at the patient's home while the patient is asleep. Nocturnal hemodialysis treatments utilize a lower blood pump flow and a longer duration of treatment time to achieve gentle treatments with better clearance of toxins and poisons.

41. When will I meet the dialysis team?

You have already met the most important member of the dialysis team. You are that person. In order to have a successful experience on dialysis, you must be an active participant in your own care. The more responsibility you take, the more information you obtain, and the more positive your attitude, the better will be your outcome on dialysis. The next member of the dialysis team that you will meet is your nephrologist. You may meet this person in his or her office, in an emergency room, in an intensive care unit, or in the dialysis unit itself. Some patients are able to meet with their doctor when they are healthy in a relaxed atmosphere. You should remember that your nephrologist has helped many patients cope with dialysis and has a great deal of experience.

If possible, it is best to meet other members of the dialysis team by visiting a dialysis unit before you begin dialysis. This will allow you to observe other patients on dialysis and talk to them about their experiences. You will spend some time talking with a senior member of the dialysis nursing team. The dialysis nurse will want to know about your medical condition. He or she will want to evaluate the access that will be used for your first dialysis. The dialysis nurse will ask you questions about your other medical conditions including any allergies, your medicines, your job, your family, and where you live, and will try to understand you as a person.

The next member of the team you will meet is the social worker. Social workers have experience helping patients adjust to dialysis. They have special training in understanding the stresses you are experiencing and can recommend strategies to help you cope with dialysis. They understand insurance companies, how to get you to dialysis and back home with transportation, and how to pay for medication. They can advise you on obtaining dialysis treatments while you are traveling or are on vacation. They pretty much tackle everything else that the other members of the team are unable to cope with. They are often the easiest member of the dialysis team to talk with. If you are having a problem, this is a good team member to approach.

You will also meet the dietitian when you visit the dialysis unit. The more I learn about medical care, the more I understand that diet is very important. Being on the right diet can be the difference between success and failure on dialysis. The dietitian has seen many patients in your situation. He or she can give you helpful hints to select the right foods to stay healthy. Many patients have foods in their culture that require expert knowledge about how much of them they can eat. Chances are your doctor will refer you to the dietitian when you have questions about what to eat.

The dialysis technicians will assist the nursing staff. They will take blood pressures, monitor the dialysis treatment, and perform many other tasks in the unit under the direction of the nurses and doctors. You may spend more time with the dialysis technicians than any other team member because they are always by your side. They tend to be caring and interested in people. They often also have a great sense of humor, which helps a lot in coping with dialysis treatments.

The dialysis unit has a team of technical support staff. These team members make sure that the water supply is safe, that the supplies are available, and are able to repair equipment at a moment's notice.

The dialysis administrator is a person who oversees the entire dialysis unit. Often the administrator will hear from other team members about problems and will be able to solve them. This person recruits staff, makes schedules, leads staff meetings, and performs a host of tasks that are often taken for granted but that are crucial to the successful running of the dialysis unit.

Being on the right diet can be the difference between success and failure on dialysis.

Preparing to Begin Dialysis

42. What will happen on my first day of hemodialysis?

Many people will feel more comfortable bringing a family member or friend with them on the first day of hemodialysis. On arrival at the hemodialysis center, you will be seated in a waiting area. A staff member will greet you and bring you into an office for a brief meeting. There are usually a few administrative tasks to complete such as filling out a data sheet of your address, telephone numbers, and emergency contact information, and you will be asked to sign a consent form giving the staff permission to treat you. A medical history and physical examination are often performed on the first day of hemodialysis. These examinations give the physician and other staff members a baseline record of your medical condition and health history, including operations, allergies, immunizations, and medications. They will also give you a chance to bring specific concerns to your doctor's attention and alert him or her to any new medical problems.

Next you will be brought by a staff member into the treatment area. Your weight will be recorded before each treatment. At your first treatment, your height will be measured. If you are beginning dialysis in a hospital hemodialysis unit, you may be placed in a bed. In most hemodialysis units, whether in or out of hospital, you will be seated in a reclining chair that has large arm rests. This chair allows the staff to change your position from seated to reclining, which is important because patients sometimes feel dizzy due to a drop in blood pressure. You will feel less dizzy when placed in a reclining position. It is also more comfortable to be able to change your position several times during the 3 to 4 hours of your treatment.

After you are seated in your reclining chair, you will notice the dialysis machine to your side. A series of tubes and an electrical wire will be going from the machine to a series of connections in the wall behind the hemodialysis machine. These tubes bring water and dialysate to the dialysis machine. Another tube brings used dialysate from the machine to a drain to be discarded. A television set is often present on the other side of your reclining chair. If you forget to bring a set of headphones, the staff may be able to lend you one.

The hemodialysis procedure begins with the staff measuring your blood pressure, pulse, and temperature. Your access will be examined. If you have a catheter, you and the staff member performing your hemodialysis will wear a mask while you are being connected to the dialysis machine. The masks are to minimize the chances of developing an infection. The staff will also perform catheter care, which involves swabbing the part of the catheter that exits the skin with an antiseptic solution to prevent infection and covering it with a clean dressing. If you have an a-v fistula or an a-v graft, it will be cleaned with an antiseptic solution such as chlorhexidine or alcohol. A staff member will insert two needles in the access and securely tape them to the skin on your arm. You are now ready to begin your first hemodialysis treatment.

The machine will begin pumping blood from one of the needles through the plastic tubing that is filled with a saline solution. This needle is called the arterial needle because blood is coming from the patient to the machine. The tubing connected to the arterial needle is color-coded red. The blood will circulate through the machine pump and into a plastic drip chamber that will allow any air in the circuit to rise to the top. It will then go through the **dialyzer,** which is a plastic cartridge that contains about 13,000 small tubes that are surrounded by dialysate. The blood will then return through the tubing to the patient through the second needle, called the venous needle. The venous needle always carries blood from the machine to the patient. The tubing connected to it is color-coded blue. Since this is your first dialysis, it may be a shorter treatment today, perhaps for 3 hours. From time to time, a blood pressure cuff attached to your arm without the a-v access will tighten as it measures your blood pressure. The alarm on your machine may go off, which means that a beeping noise begins with a flashing light on the machine. This alarm does not indicate danger. It is designed to alert the staff to some parameter that needs checking.

As you look around, you will see other patients coming into the unit to begin their dialysis treatment. Other patients will be chatting with the person next to them or with staff members. Some patients will be sleeping, watching television, or reading a book. Other patients will be finishing their treatment and weighing themselves. After your dialysis treatment is finished, your weight, blood pressure, pulse, and temperature are recorded and are useful pieces of information to be used when you return for your next treatment. Staff members will be checking on you during your treatment. They may ask you for information or try to teach you some of the important points about the dialysis treatment. Do not expect to absorb too much

Dialyzer

A medical device that contains the dialysis membrane. It is connected to tubing that allows blood to flow into the dialyzer on one side of the membrane and then back to the patient. Dialysate flows on the other side of the membrane, and poisons and toxins move from the blood across the membrane into the dialysate, which is then discarded.

information on your first treatment. After your pre-scribed dialysis time is completed, an alarm (a beeping noise) will sound. The staff will flush the plastic tubing with saline solution. The lines will then be clamped, and the tubing will be disconnected from the needles. One needle will be removed, and a sterile gauze will be held over the needle hole with firm pressure until the bleeding has stopped. A Band-Aid will then be applied over the needle hole. The second needle will then be removed. It is a good idea to get up slowly after your dialysis treatment. Because fluid has been removed, patients can sometimes feel a bit dizzy. Do not forget to weigh yourself after your treatment. You will return for your next treatment in 2 days. Perhaps for your next treatment you will bring something to read or your iPod to listen to your favorite music to help pass the time.

43. How will I begin my peritoneal dialysis?

Peritoneal dialysis begins with the insertion of the peritoneal dialysis catheter. This access is a flexible plastic tube that is inserted into the abdomen during a minor surgical procedure under local anesthesia with sedation. The procedure is usually done as an outpa-tient. You may not have to stay overnight. A dressing or bandage will cover the incision as well as the catheter. It will take about 2 weeks for your catheter to heal before it can be used. This time will be spent learning how to perform your peritoneal dialysis. Peri-toneal dialysis is a home dialysis procedure, but your training will take place at the peritoneal dialysis unit. The unit may be located in a hemodialysis center or

Peritoneal dialysis is a home dialysis procedure, but your training will take place at the peritoneal dialysis unit.

may be in or close to a hospital or doctor's office. Most units have videos, slide shows, and printed material that will be used in your training. During the healing of your catheter, the peritoneal dialysis nurse or your physician may flush the catheter with a saline solution to keep the catheter from becoming clogged.

When your peritoneal dialysis catheter is ready, you will come to the peritoneal dialysis unit for training. After washing your hands, you will put on a face mask to prevent bacteria from your mouth and nose becoming aerosolized and landing on the catheter while it is being connected to tubing. Your peritoneal dialysis nurse will show you how to connect your catheter to plastic tubing. This task is not very hard, but it will take some time to feel comfortable performing it. The tubing is connected to a plastic bag containing 2 liters of peritoneal dialysis solution. This solution will be placed above your abdomen on a pole similar to those used for intravenous solutions in hospitals (**Figure 5**). A clamp will be opened to allow the peritoneal dialysis fluid to gently run into your abdomen. After the plastic bag is empty, you will disconnect the plastic tubing. The catheter will be secured to your abdomen with a dressing or an elastic belt. You are now free to walk around, eat, read, or perform any of the many activities that you normally would participate in during the day. When it is time to drain the fluid from your abdomen, you will again wash your hands and put on your face mask. After connecting your catheter to the plastic tubing, you will open the clamp and let the solution in your abdomen drain out into an empty plastic bag placed on the floor. The fluid from the abdomen flows out because of gravity. After the abdomen is emptied, the new peritoneal dialysis fluid will be hung on the

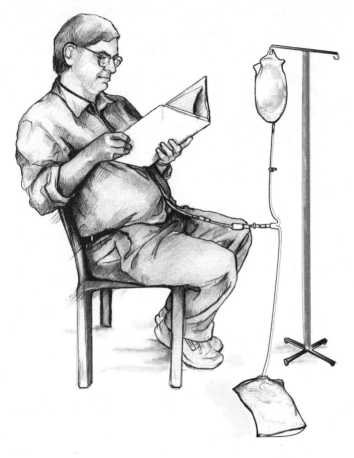

Figure 5   A peritoneal dialysis patient

Source: National Institute of Diabetes and Digestive and Kidney Diseases, National Institutes of Health.

Exchange

A term used in peritoneal dialysis that describes fluid being drained using plastic tubing from the abdomen into a collection bag. New peritoneal dialysate is infused by gravity into the abdomen.

pole to allow flow into the abdomen. The used peritoneal dialysis fluid containing poisons and waste products is then discarded down the drain of a sink. This process of emptying the abdomen of dialysate and refilling the abdomen with fresh dialysate is called an **exchange**. The peritoneal dialysis exchange is not painful. Most patients perform 4 exchanges a day.

Peritoneal dialysis training usually takes place Monday through Friday. You may also be receiving hemodialysis treatments during your training to remove the toxins and waste products until you can perform the exchanges. As part of your peritoneal dialysis training, you will learn how to inject medications into the peritoneal dialysis bag. You will also learn to recognize the signs and symptoms of infection of the abdomen called peritonitis. Nutritional information will be given to you to help you choose healthy foods. The peritoneal dialysis training takes approximately 2 weeks for most people. Some patients learn faster than others. The most important point is to feel comfortable doing the dialysis. When you are confident with your peritoneal dialysis technique, the nurse will arrange for your supplies to be delivered to your home. After your training is completed, you will visit the peritoneal dialysis unit every month. The peritoneal dialysis nurse will check your catheter and draw monthly blood tests. You will review your progress with your physician at this visit. If problems occur between visits, a nurse is available by telephone 24 hours a day. You can contact the nurse who may direct you to come to the peritoneal dialysis unit or give you advice over the telephone.

PART FOUR

Living Well on Dialysis

Since beginning dialysis, I feel tired all the time. Will this improve with time?

Can dialysis patients be sexually active?

Can I travel as a dialysis patient?

More ...

44. Will my friends and family be able to tell I am on dialysis?

Even though I have special training in nephrology, I often cannot tell that people I meet in social situations are on dialysis. In the early days of dialysis, the dialysis was very inefficient in removing waste products and toxins. Patients were pale and had sickly looking complexions. It was common to smell an odor of urea caused by the very high levels of urea in the blood. Patients had severe deformities of the bones caused by metabolic bone disease. Patients today on dialysis are completely different. Modern hemodialysis and peritoneal dialysis are much more efficient at removing toxins and poisons from the blood. Less of these toxins present means there are less deposited in the skin. Erythropoietin is administered to most patients with anemia to raise their red blood cell count. The pale sickly complexion is not present in most patients. Patients are stronger because of their higher red blood cell count and have a much greater exercise tolerance. Because they look and feel better, they do not act like sick people. Of course, everyone is different. Some patients have severe systemic illnesses like hardening of the arteries, poorly-controlled diabetes, lupus erythematosus, or kidney failure associated with cancer. These individuals will appear ill.

The presence of a hemodialysis access in the arm is a tip off that a person is on hemodialysis. The access does not bother most patients. They leave the arm uncovered or wear long sleeves so the access is less noticeable. Some patients will discuss the placement of the access with their vascular surgeon. An a-v access in the upper arm may be less noticeable and is preferred by some patients.

One of the tricks to help you do well on dialysis is paying a little more attention to your appearance. It is important to comb and style your hair, wear a favorite shirt, or dress up a little. Women receiving dialysis treatments will often put on their makeup and tasteful jewelry before they come to their treatment. If you look good, people are less likely to respond to you as a sick person. You will feel better about yourself, have more self-esteem, and transmit these feelings to others who in turn will relate to you in a more positive way. Try this approach and see if it works for you.

If you look good, people are less likely to respond to you as a sick person.

I encourage people to tell their family, friends, and close colleagues at work that they are receiving dialysis treatments. This will give you additional people to talk with about problems. Many times, these people are sources of support. They may volunteer to drive you to dialysis when your car breaks down, help cover you at work when you have a doctor's appointment, and understand why you are having an occasional rough day. People you are close to may sense that you are sick from your actions. Many times people assume you have a worse condition than you actually have. Most of us know people who are on dialysis and are very accepting of the need for dialysis treatments.

45. Since beginning dialysis, I feel tired all the time. Will this improve with time?

Energy levels vary among individuals both before and after starting dialysis. We all know people who are in constant motion. They work hard, find time for a variety of activities and hobbies, and are always ready to go off on another endeavor at a moment's notice. The rest of us feel tired just thinking about doing these things. It is important to realize that dialysis is physically and psychologically demanding. You should take extra care of yourself during the stage when you are beginning dialysis treatments. You should get a full night's sleep. Make sure you sit down and eat three meals a day and a snack even though you are not hungry. It is also wise to avoid extra stress in your life like changing where you live, taking on a new job, or divorcing your spouse. These experiences can take a lot out of you and add to your fatigue.

The first thing to do if you feel tired is to review your medications with your physician. Many medications for blood pressure and pain, and some ulcer medications called histamine H_2-receptor antagonists, have side effects that will make you tired. Patients on dialysis are more likely to have side effects from medications, possibly because they metabolize medications more slowly than patients with normal renal function. Sleeping pills can build up in your body over time and cause you to be tired. Medications prescribed for anxiety and depression can sometimes decrease your energy level.

Because kidney failure causes our sleep-wake cycle to be reversed, many patients with kidney failure have difficulty sleeping at night. Patients may instead fall asleep during the day. This problem is due to changes in the body's hormonal cycle. Better sleep at night can be achieved by avoiding naps during the day. It is a good idea not to drink caffeinated beverages in the hours preceding sleep.

46. Can dialysis patients be sexually active?

Yes. There is nothing about hemodialysis or peritoneal dialysis treatments that would interfere with sexual activity. An interest in and the ability to engage in sexual activity is a sign of good health in kidney dialysis patients.

Some dialysis patients worry that sexual activity will damage their dialysis access. In hemodialysis, an a-v fistula or graft is usually located in the arm and is not affected by sexual activity. A hemodialysis catheter should be protected with a clean sterile dressing that is securely taped to the patient's chest. The peritoneal dialysis access is a catheter located in the lower abdomen. A clean, securely taped dressing over the catheter is all that is needed to protect it during sexual intercourse.

Recent research has discovered that the inability to participate in sexual intercourse in men with erectile dysfunction predicts their cardiac disease. Patients need to have a good vascular system so that blood can travel to the sexual organs as well as the heart. Smoking, poorly-controlled diabetes, high blood pressure, and an elevated cholesterol level can lead to hardening of the arteries. This process, called atherosclerosis, causes blockages in blood vessels all over the body. As a dialysis patient, you may have one or more of these conditions. It is important to decrease your risk of developing atherosclerosis to preserve your sexual function. The most important measure you can take to remain sexually active as you age is to stop smoking.

An interest in and the ability to engage in sexual activity is a sign of good health in kidney dialysis patients.

Living Well on Dialysis

Another major cause of sexual problems in dialysis patients is neuropathy. Neuropathy is damage to the peripheral nerves that exit the spinal cord and go to our arms, legs, skin, blood vessels, sexual organs, and other parts of our body. Poisons and toxins that build up in our blood in kidney failure can cause this nerve damage. Neuropathy can be prevented by having effective dialysis treatments to remove these substances. It is important that your dialysis treatment remove as much poisons and toxins as possible. This means a longer dialysis treatment. The longer we stay on dialysis, the more toxins and poisons are removed. Other causes of neuropathy in dialysis patients include poorly-controlled diabetes, alcohol abuse, vitamin B_{12} and thiamine deficiency, hypothyroidism, HIV/AIDS infection, vasculitis, and amyloidosis.

Medications can interfere with sexual activity. Many of the first blood pressure medications interfered with sexual activity, especially in men. Most of the new blood pressure medications are free of this unfortunate side effect. Medications for depression, anxiety, and sleeping pills can cause a decrease in interest in sexual activity.

If you have concerns about your sexual function, it is important to discuss this with your doctor in private. As a dialysis patient, many of your interactions with your doctor will be in the dialysis unit where there are other patients and staff members present, which is not the best place to discuss your concerns. Many patients are uncomfortable talking about sexual matters. Many doctors are also somewhat uncomfortable. It is a good idea to ask for a meeting in private and indicate why you wish to meet to allow your doctor to think about your case, review your medications, and develop an approach to working with you on your sexual health. You may or may not want to bring your spouse or sexual partner to the meeting. This is up to you.

The approach to treating kidney patients on dialysis with sexual problems is similar to treating patients who are not on dialysis. The evaluation and therapies are the same. If your dialysis physician is unable to treat your problem, he or she may refer you to a physician with special expertise in this field. Traditionally urologists have developed an interest in treating sexual problems. Gynecologists are often a good resource for women. It is important to find a physician with whom you feel comfortable discussing your sexual health in a nonjudgmental way.

Erick Lucero writes:

I began dialysis suddenly after my blood tests took a turn for the worse. At the time, I was tired and depressed. I didn't have much energy. I had a procedure to insert a catheter into my neck and another operation to put an a–v fistula in my arm. My doctor didn't talk to me about sex. My wife also had questions. At first, I was afraid that sexual activity would make me feel worse. After a month on dialysis, my wife and I decided on our own to have sex.

Since beginning dialysis, I feel better and have a lot more energy. My wife and I have sex more often. We use birth control because we are not ready to have another child. I feel that a discussion about when it is advisable to begin sexual activity should be part of the protocol of every patient's counseling about beginning dialysis. This would be really helpful to patients.

47. Can I have children while I am being treated with dialysis?

Men who have kidney failure can father children. Women have difficulty becoming pregnant. This is because many women with kidney failure stop menstruating. They do not release eggs from their ovaries. If they do have menstrual periods, they often have anovulatory cycles. This means that they do not release an egg cell from their ovaries. When women do have a normal period and become pregnant, the fertilized egg has difficulty developing normally, and there is an increased chance of a spontaneous miscarriage. Despite these limitations, a few women become pregnant on dialysis. As dialysis becomes more efficient and patients have higher blood counts due to erythropoietin, it is possible for more women to become pregnant on dialysis. Very few of these pregnancies are successful. Many of the babies are born too early and are premature.

It is important for women on dialysis to discuss their medical condition with their obstetrician-gynecologist. There may be medical reasons why becoming pregnant might be dangerous to a woman's health. If you think you might be pregnant, it is important to tell your physician. Your physician can review your medications to determine which ones are safe in pregnancy. ACE inhibiters and angiotensin receptor blockers used for treating high blood pressure and heart failure should be stopped if you could be pregnant. These drugs can cause a miscarriage. If you are on these medications, do not panic. Many women on these medications have had successful pregnancies after conceiving. Your doctor can guide you in selecting other medications that are safe for pregnancy. Some birth control methods may be safer than others for women with kidney failure.

Women on birth control pills have a higher chance of stroke and clots that can form in their legs. Birth control methods such as condoms and the diaphragm are well tolerated and safe for dialysis patients. Ask your kidney physician which method is right for you. Women who receive kidney transplants have a very rapid return to fertility and could conceive in the first month after receiving their transplant. Patients are most likely to reject their new kidney during the first 2 years of their transplant. Women need to receive counseling on avoiding becoming pregnant during this important time. After 2 years, if all is going well with the kidney transplant, your transplant physician will advise you that it is safe to become pregnant. Kidney transplantation is the best option for women with kidney failure who want to have a family.

Erick Lucero writes:

I got married before I began hemodialysis treatments. I thought my life was over, and I would be bedridden and sick. My wife was very supportive. She encouraged me to get married despite having renal failure. We planned the pregnancy together. One year before beginning dialysis, we had a beautiful baby girl. My daughter helps me a lot by taking my mind off of dialysis. When I started dialysis, I took time off from work and would take her to the park. She is the best.

Since beginning dialysis, we have thought about having another child, but we are not ready yet. We use birth control and will plan on when to have the next baby. I am worried about the finances of having another child. Also my wife does most of the child care because I am at work or on dialysis. It is easy to take care of one baby, but two with one parent during the day will be harder.

48. How long can I live on dialysis?

This is the most frequent question I am asked by patients who are beginning dialysis. Patients who do not ask this important question must be thinking about it. Doctors developed the ability to treat large numbers of patients with chronic kidney failure in the 1970s. The technology to treat these patients with dialysis was poor. The machines were inaccurate. Doctors could not remove large amounts of poisons and toxins. Medications to treat anemia, hypertension, high cholesterol, diabetes, and heart disease were not as effective as modern medications. Despite these limitations, some patients were able to live for over 30 years after beginning dialysis. Patients beginning dialysis today benefit from better dialysis treatments, better medications, better nursing and medical care, and an expectation by the medical community that they will do well on dialysis. In the 1970s, many physicians felt there was no point in treating patients with dialysis because the prognosis was so poor. This attitude has disappeared as doctors began to see long-term survivors on dialysis. Dialysis will continue to improve due to new discoveries and advances in technology. The major causes of death in the United States and other developed countries are heart disease, stroke, and cancer. The outlook for these diseases is rapidly improving and will continue to improve. Improved treatment of these other diseases will also lead to patients living longer on dialysis.

Patients beginning dialysis today benefit from better dialysis treatments, better medications, better nursing and medical care, and an expectation by the medical community that they will do well on dialysis.

It is hard to answer patients who want to know how long they will live. Doctors do not know the answer to this crucial question. There is no reason why a highly motivated patient with no other serious medical conditions who began dialysis at 20 years of age could not live for 50 years or more on dialysis. What do I mean by a highly motivated patient? There are four goals that every patient must accomplish to live a long life on dialysis:

1. You must achieve a good dialysis. This does not mean just removing lots of fluid. It means that a large amount of poisons and toxins must be removed. To accomplish this, you must have a good dialysis access. You must have enough time on dialysis. If you are on hemodialysis, this probably means at least 4 hours of hemodialysis 3 times a week. You must not skip any dialysis treatments or fail to perform peritoneal dialysis exchanges. Your healthcare team will be meeting with you and discussing with you the adequacy of your dialysis.

2. You must take special care to keep on your diet and fluid restriction. The more we learn about illness, we realize that what we eat and drink is very important. Patients who continually eat and drink inappropriate foods to excess will decrease their chances of being long-term survivors on dialysis.

3. Make sure you always take your medication. Having a high blood pressure, elevated blood sugar if you are a diabetic, elevated cholesterol, or bone disease will take its toll over the years.

4. Listen to common sense advice concerning your health. This means not smoking, drinking to excess, or using drugs. It means wearing your seatbelt and not driving too fast. If you are a biker or skier, it means wearing a helmet. If you have a gun, keep it locked up and away from children. Do not swim alone. These measures are important for you and your family whether you are treated with dialysis or not.

49. Can I shorten my dialysis treatments?

Patients, doctors, and nurses have always been interested in decreasing the amount of time on dialysis. Patients want to spend as little time on dialysis as possible. It is difficult to sit in one place for 4 hours. The last hour of dialysis is physically and mentally difficult for some patients. A hemodialysis treatment which would last 3 hours or 2½ hours would be much easier than a 4- or 5-hour dialysis treatment.

To accomplish this, high-flux (or high-efficiency) hemodialysis was developed during the 1980s. The blood flow running through the dialysis machine was increased from 300 mL/min to 450 mL/min. Large dialysis membranes with large surface areas were used to allow more blood to be in contact with more dialysate. Dialysis times were decreased to 3, 2½, and sometimes even 2¼ hours. The owners of dialysis units were encouraged by high-flux dialysis because less hours for dialysis meant less nursing labor costs. The results of the experiment with high-flux dialysis were a disaster. Patients had more complications. Patients treated with high-flux dialysis did not live as long as patients on regular, longer dialysis. High-flux dialysis was abandoned, and patients went back to longer dialysis treatments.

Several important lessons were learned from this experiment. The importance of increasing blood flow to achieve better removal of poisons and toxins was recognized. The need for better dialyzers with increased clearances and surface areas was appreciated. This finding allowed regular, longer dialysis treatments to remove more poisons and toxins, which made dialysis better by decreasing complications of kidney failure such as neuropathy. In the early days of dialysis, many patients suffered from pericarditis (an inflammation of the lining of the heart). Patients accumulated fluid in the lung called pleural effusion, or in the abdomen called ascites. These complications are much less frequent now that dialysis is more efficient and removes more toxins.

Recently, nocturnal hemodialysis has allowed patients to receive dialysis treatments 6 nights a week while they sleep. This home dialysis treatment involves hemodialysis with a low blood flow rate for 6 to 7 hours, 6 nights a week. Patients have much more toxins and poisons removed with this increased dialysis time and feel better. They are able to eat more varieties of food containing potassium and phosphorus that are restricted in the diet of patients on dialysis three times a week. Fluid restriction is not necessary because of daily fluid removal. Blood pressure is decreased by nocturnal dialysis, and some patients can decrease or stop their blood pressure medications. The present trend is to increase the time on dialysis to improve patient outcomes. The best way to decrease time on dialysis is to consider a kidney transplant. This will allow you to stop dialysis completely.

50. Can I travel as a dialysis patient?

Since the 1970s, patients and doctors on dialysis have been trying to overcome the psychological effects of being connected to the hemodialysis machine. Early on, there were few dialysis centers and travel was limited. Several doctors developed miniature portable hemodialysis machines that were set up by the patient and allowed them to travel. These machines never really caught on, though. One problem is water quality. All modern dialysis centers have an extensive water purification system, which consists of a series of filters to remove particulate matter. After passing through these filters, the water is pumped at high pressure through a reverse osmosis membrane to eliminate elements such as aluminum and copper, producing water that is pure. Reverse osmosis membranes and filters are available for home use, but they significantly increase the size of the dialysis machine. This makes traveling with your dialysis machine difficult. There are dialysis systems that regenerate dialysis and do not require large amounts of pure water. Recently, a new machine called the Nx Stage, which is simpler to set up and use, has become available.

Many hemodialysis units will admit patients that travel who are known as transient patients.

As more hemodialysis centers opened, the need for portable dialysis machines that could be taken with the patient decreased. Many hemodialysis units will admit patients that travel who are known as transient patients. You must plan ahead. Arranging for hemodialysis at another center is best done several months before your trip. Most units will require you to send part of your medical record, which includes a copy of your last physical examination and blood tests. Some centers will want a chest x-ray, **EKG**, and HIV testing before they will accept you. Most centers are happy to have you dialyze with them. They realize that their own patients will travel and know that a warm welcome to transient patients will make their trip successful.

Electrocardiogram (EKG)

A medical test in which electrical impulses generated by the heart are recorded by attaching electrodes to the arms, legs, and chest.

Your health insurance will pay for dialysis treatments within the United States. If you want to travel to another country, you will probably have to pay for the treatments. This can be expensive, up to $600 per treatment at some European dialysis units. Some cruise ship lines have organized cruises for dialysis patients. The ship will have hemodialysis machines as well as doctors and nurses on board to allow you to receive your treatments. They will also arrange to serve meals that are healthy for renal patients. One of the difficulties in traveling is the temptation to go off the renal diet because food that is low in sodium, potassium, and phosphorus is harder to find.

Patients on peritoneal dialysis have an easier time traveling. They can arrange to have supplies shipped to their travel destination and do not have to depend on a dialysis unit because they perform their own treatment. They have more flexibility and can change their itinerary at a moment's notice. This is one of the benefits of peritoneal dialysis treatments.

51. Is home dialysis for me?

Home dialysis has many important advantages to the patient. Because home dialysis patients usually perform their own dialysis treatment, they learn a great deal about how to effectively treat kidney failure. The home dialysis patient is able to schedule his or her treatments around work and family responsibilities and has the flexibility to perform an extra treatment if needed. There is no travel time to the dialysis center, which is especially important for patients who live in rural areas who would have to travel several hours to the nearest dialysis center. In some parts of the world, there are no dialysis units, and home dialysis or kidney transplant are the only option. Some patients must leave their country to obtain dialysis treatments. They cannot go back home because dialysis is not available on many of the Caribbean Islands or in some parts of South America, Africa, and Asia. This is rapidly changing. Many countries are developing dialysis centers to offer modern treatments to their citizens. Home dialysis is cheaper. The cost of the dialysis is the supplies and dialysis machine. There is no cost for the person performing the dialysis, as the patient is doing the work. There is no rent for the dialysis unit, no heating or air conditioning costs, insurance costs, or extra telephone service. Patients on home dialysis do not have to wait their turn to begin their treatment.

The disadvantages of home dialysis are few. Some patients feel more comfortable in the dialysis center because their doctor will see them while they are receiving hemodialysis. Dialysis nurses and technicians will perform your hemodialysis at the dialysis unit. Most patients on home dialysis perform their own dialysis treatment. On home dialysis, you will go to the doctor's office once a month. The dialysis team may make a home visit, but for the most part you will be on dialysis at home with your **dialysis partner**. My colleague and friend Dr. Roxanna Bologa, Director of Peritoneal Dialysis at the Rogosin Institute, tells her patients, "Just because you are on home dialysis does not mean you are alone." Your doctor and nurse are just a phone call away.

Dialysis partner

A person who has received special training in performing hemodialysis or peritoneal dialysis and who assists you in performing dialysis at home.

Most patients on home hemodialysis have a family member help them with their dialysis. A few home hemodialysis patients have a nurse or dialysis technician perform their dialysis at home. Most insurances will not pay for a dialysis nurse at home. Peritoneal dialysis patients usually perform their own treatment at home. Some elderly patients or children have the dialysis performed by a family member.

Many hemodialysis patients begin hemodialysis treatments at the dialysis unit under the care of their doctors and nurses. When they feel comfortable on dialysis, they begin training with a partner and learn to perform their own dialysis. These patients then dialyze at home. If their medical condition changes, they can always go back to the dialysis unit for a period of time when they may need closer observation. The best way to determine if home dialysis is for you is to talk with patients on home dialysis. They can give firsthand information about dialysis at home and share some of their experiences with you.

52. Will dialysis frighten my young children?

Children are very adaptable. They are perceptive and can sense when adults are hiding things from them to "protect them." Children are exposed to many different kinds of illness by the media. Human-interest stories on television and the newspapers have graphic pictures of patients with all sorts of medical conditions, including kidney failure. News reports show dead bodies of people who have died by illness, natural disasters, or wars. I am amazed that it is common to view actual operations on daytime television that can be seen by young children. The best approach with your children is to explain to them that you have a kidney problem and that your dialysis treatments will help you remain healthy. Explain to them when you will be having your dialysis treatments and when you will be away from home. The amount of information you give your child will of course depend on your child's age. Teenagers may better understand the scientific aspects of dialysis.

The best approach with your children is to explain to them that you have a kidney problem and that your dialysis treatments will help you remain healthy.

It is best not to take young children into the dialysis unit. Young children could be potentially distracting to the dialysis caregivers who should focus on giving you the best possible dialysis treatment and not be worried about the effect on your child of seeing a parent on dialysis. Having your child keep you company while you are on home dialysis is fine. It is a good time to talk, watch television together, or perhaps review a homework assignment. It is reasonable to have your child visit you if you are hospitalized. In general, it is better if children avoid going to the intensive care unit. They may be exposed to infectious diseases carried by other patients, and the experience of seeing critically ill patients may be upsetting.

I find that older adult children are much more disturbed by a parent on dialysis than are younger children. They are much more fearful that dialysis will mean they will lose you to illness. A good way to cope with these fears is to assign your children tasks to help you. Have them bring your favorite sweater or book to the hospital. Let them drive you to the dialysis unit or to doctors' visits. This involvement will allow them to adjust to seeing you on dialysis and will make them less fearful. It will give you both time to talk about the impact kidney dialysis is having on your life. It is important not to underestimate the impact of your kidney failure and dialysis treatments on your family. Even though you are doing well and are making progress, this is a major stress for your spouse, children, significant other, and friends. Talk about the impact of your dialysis treatment on your family with your doctor and the dialysis team. Your doctor has seen hundreds of patients and their families cope with kidney dialysis. You have the experience of one person.

53. Can I drive my car to my dialysis treatments?

Many patients drive to their dialysis treatments. You should absolutely not drive your car to your first dialysis treatment. You will be under a great deal of stress, and you will need to have someone else get you to dialysis and get you home. Driving to dialysis is not a problem. Driving home after your treatment is more of a concern. During the hemodialysis treatment, 2 to 3 liters of fluid (a little less than 2 to 3 quarts) are removed from your blood. Sometimes this can cause your blood pressure to decrease, and you might feel a bit weak or dizzy after your dialysis treatment. This effect is especially common during the first few weeks on hemodialysis. I generally counsel patients to arrange for 2 weeks of transportation when beginning hemodialysis. Some insurance plans will pay for transportation to and from the dialysis unit. After this time, you can ask your doctor if he or she feels it is safe for you to drive to your treatments. Having kidney dialysis treatments will make you eligible for a handicapped parking permit. Talk to your dialysis social worker who can help you obtain this useful permit.

Erick Lucero writes:

When I first started dialysis, I didn't want to drive to my treatments. I had a new a-v fistula in my arm, and I felt I needed two strong arms to drive safely. After several weeks, I began to drive to my dialysis treatments. Parking can be a problem near my dialysis unit. I have a metrocard in my pocket for emergencies. If I cannot find a parking spot I park at home and take the bus to the dialysis unit. I'm not far away—about 10 blocks. I can walk to dialysis if I have to. After working all day and being on dialysis for 4 hours, I want to be home as soon as possible.

54. What can I do during my dialysis treatments?

Your hemodialysis treatment will last $3\frac{1}{2}$ to 4 hours. Part of this time will be spent talking to the dialysis staff to tell them how you are feeling, checking your blood pressure and temperature, and having any needed prescriptions refilled by your doctor. You will use your time on dialysis to talk to the dietitian to learn which foods are healthy for you to eat and which foods are best avoided. Your nurse and physician will review your medications and let you know how your dialysis treatments are going. The social worker will visit with you from time to time. Our dialysis unit has a **podiatrist** and a psychologist who will see patients while they are on hemodialysis treatment. This allows them to use their days off hemodialysis for other activities.

Podiatrist

A healthcare professional who is trained in the diagnosis and treatment of disorders of the feet.

Patients look forward to chatting with other patients in the waiting area of the dialysis unit and during hemodialysis treatments. They exchange experiences and support each other during difficult times. Many patients on the same dialysis shift have their treatments at the same time for several years, and there is a social aspect to the dialysis unit that is enjoyable. Some patients, especially patients who work full time, take the opportunity to nap. If you work 40 hours a week and have dialysis 4 hours, 3 times a week, using your time on dialysis to catch up on your rest is a good strategy. The laptop computer has enabled many patients to get their work done while on dialysis. Teachers often spend their time on dialysis grading papers or working on lesson plans. Watching television is always an option. Every dialysis unit has televisions, usually personal flat screen units that are provided free. Bring your headphones. If you forget them, the unit may be able to lend you a pair. It is common to see patients watching movies on DVD players or laptops. Libraries will lend you DVDs and books on CD or tapes. Did I forget to mention reading books? Some patients will bring their Bible or religious reading material to dialysis. Take your time enjoying the newspaper. Read that catalogue of fishing equipment laying on your desk at home. Consider learning a new language on DVD or tape. College lectures are also available to listen to and watch. Crossword puzzles, word puzzles, and sudoku are very popular. Most dialysis units allow you to talk on your cell phone. Call your nephew to see how he is doing in his first year of college. Catch up with old friends. You may need to increase the minutes on you calling plan when you begin dialysis. Patients use their time on dialysis to work on knitting and crochet. One of my patients on hemodialysis is presently knitting beautiful wool hats.

Patients on peritoneal dialysis spend most of their time performing their exchanges. It takes about 20 minutes to drain the fluid from their abdomen and another 20 minutes to infuse the fresh dialysate. This time can be spent doing other activities.

One approach to hemodialysis treatments is to resent every minute you are forced to spend on dialysis. Another approach is to find activities that are useful and productive, either from a recreational or work point of view (**Figure 6**). Remember, dialysis is the perfect excuse for finding some time for you.

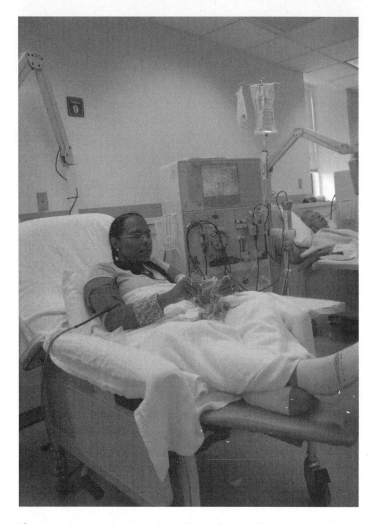

Figure 6   A patient, Yoshi Reynolds, crocheting during her hemodialysis treatment
Source: K. Neelakantappa, MD

55. Will I have the same nurse or technician for every hemodialysis treatment?

Most patients develop close relationships with the members of the dialysis team that take care of them three times a week. It is natural to trust these skilled caregivers and to feel threatened if they are not always available. Team members call in sick, go on vacation, or have responsibilities at home that may make them unavailable for your dialysis treatment. Because no team member can be available all the time, it is common to rotate the dialysis staff within the dialysis unit. This allows a larger number of staff members to be familiar with your treatment. Some patients have difficulty with inserting needles into their dialysis access. There is always one staff member in every unit who is especially skilled at placing dialysis needles. This procedure is called **cannulation** of the access. It is important that staff members in the unit communicate with other staff members about your access. This way, a variety of staff members will be able to place you on dialysis if your regular nurse or technician is not available. Some patients have a fall in blood pressure at the same time during their hemodialysis treatment. Staff members who know this will be able to give you some extra fluid at the right time to prevent you from getting dizzy or sick. As you spend more time on dialysis, you will have less anxiety about new staff members performing your dialysis. Feel free to give them helpful advice about your particular pattern on hemodialysis.

Most patients develop close relationships with the members of the dialysis team that take care of them three times a week.

Cannulation

The insertion of needles into the dialysis access to obtain blood for hemodialysis.

56. Which vaccines should I receive?

When you begin your dialysis treatments, you will be tested for hepatitis B as well as hepatitis C. A series of three immunizations is available to stimulate antibody production by your body against hepatitis B. These antibodies will decrease your chances of developing hepatitis B if you are exposed. Most patients who do not have antibodies decide to receive the hepatitis B vaccine. Vaccination is also available for hepatitis A, but protection only lasts for about 6 months. This vaccine is useful if you will be traveling to areas that have a large number of hepatitis A cases. If you have chronic hepatitis C, you should take the hepatitis B vaccine to prevent further damage to your liver.

Patients on dialysis are offered the pneumococcal vaccine. This can protect you from developing pneumococcal pneumonia. This potentially life-threatening illness can be more serious in dialysis and kidney transplant patients because their immune response to infection is decreased by kidney failure. The anti-rejection medications taken by kidney transplant patients also decrease the body's defense against infection. I always recommend the influenza vaccine to my patients and coworkers at the dialysis unit. Being sick with the flu is no fun. You can transmit influenza virus to members of your family and other people. The risks are small compared to the benefits. Kidney dialysis patients should receive the inactivated influenza vaccine. They should not receive the live attenuated influenza vaccine. Hepatitis B vaccine, pneumococcal vaccine, and the inactivated influenza vaccine are routinely given to patients in the dialysis unit. As part of your dialysis evaluation, you will have a skin test for tuberculosis. In some countries, the **BCG** vaccine is given to patients to prevent tuberculosis. BCG is not recommended for patients in the United States. For more information, the Center for Disease Control and Prevention has prepared Guidelines for Vaccination in Kidney Dialysis Patients and Patients with Chronic Kidney Diseases (*www.cdc.gov*).

BCG

Bacillus Calmette-Guerin is a tuberculosis vaccine given to children in many countries with a high prevalence of tuberculosis. Patients who have received BCG will often have a positive skin test for tuberculosis for the rest of their lives.

PART FIVE

Nutrition on Dialysis

Why do I have to watch what I eat?

What is a renal diet?

Why are potassium and phosphorus so important?

More ...

Most physicians have a registered dietitian working with them in the dialysis center who can refine your dietary plan and give you specific information regarding the nutritional content of foods.

57. Why do I have to watch what I eat?

As we learn more about the science of medical illness, we realize that diet is very important. As a kidney dialysis patient, you will need expert advice regarding your own individual diet. Many well-meaning people will give you advice, urging you to drink more fluid to flush your kidneys, or to drink cranberry juice. Thank these well wishers for their concern, then discuss your diet with your physician. He or she may not be able to give you all the answers you need, but you will be pointed in the right direction. Your physician can guide you to eat more calories if you need to gain weight or restrict calories to lose weight. He or she will know how much fluid intake is advisable and which foods to avoid if you have high cholesterol, diabetes, heart problems, or other medical conditions. Most physicians have a registered dietitian working with them in the dialysis center who can refine your dietary plan and give you specific information regarding the nutritional content of foods. The dietitian will work with you to help you choose foods that you will like to eat and that are good for you.

Edema

The medical term for fluid that collects in an area of the body. The most common location for edema is in the legs. The legs appear swollen, especially after walking around. The edema decreases after a night's sleep because it has moved to other areas of the body. Other areas that can collect fluid are the lungs and abdomen.

If our kidneys are normal, we are able to eat a large variety of foods without a thought. If we eat a large amount of salt, our kidneys will measure the increase and immediately take steps to begin eliminating the salt from our body. If we drink a large amount of fluid, our kidneys will recognize this fluid overload and begin increasing urine formation. If our kidneys become damaged, they lose their ability to respond to variations in diet. Often, diseased kidneys begin retaining salt and fluid when they should be eliminating them. This fluid and salt retention can cause swelling of our legs. The medical term for this is **edema**. As we retain more fluid and salt, some of the fluid can back up into our lungs and cause shortness of breath. Fluid retention will also cause our blood pressure to rise and be uncontrolled. This is why kidney patients must measure and restrict the amount of fluid and salt they consume every day.

Once we begin our dialysis treatments, fluid, salt, and other substances are removed during the dialysis treatment. If we are on hemodialysis, about 2 to 3 liters are removed during each treatment. This is about 2.1 to 3.2 quarts of fluid. Removing more fluid on hemodialysis is not that easy or comfortable for the patient. Therefore, it would be advisable to limit fluid intake to the amount we can safely remove. If we are on hemodialysis every other day, this means decreasing our intake to 1 to 1.5 liters a day. Our kidneys no longer can tell that we are gaining fluid. We can tell by weighing ourselves. If we drink 1 liter of fluid, our weight increases by 2.2 pounds. Hemodialysis patients routinely weigh themselves before and after their treatments to see if they have had a successful treatment. Peritoneal dialysis patients weigh themselves every day. Because peritoneal dialysis patients are on dialysis every day, they can often drink more fluid than hemodialysis patients on a daily basis. If they drink too much, and their weight increases, they can increase the amount of fluid removed by changing the dialysate. This ability to remove fluid and salt on a daily basis is one of the advantages of peritoneal dialysis.

While on kidney dialysis, you will be constantly monitoring the levels of potassium, phosphorus, calcium, and cholesterol in your blood. These tests will be measured on a monthly basis, and you will receive a copy of your blood test results and discuss these findings with the dialysis team. If you are a diabetic, you will also monitor your glucose or sugar level on a daily basis. By making small changes in your diet in response to these blood tests, you can improve your results. This seems like a lot of work, but patients will spend a great deal of time learning about diet when they begin dialysis. As time goes on, they will become more accustomed to their diet and will have an easier time making healthy food choices.

58. What is a renal diet?

Renal diet

A diet that avoids foods that contain sodium, potassium, and phosphorus, and limits the amount of fluid intake.

A **renal diet** is a term used to describe the guidelines developed for patients with renal disease. Your dietitian and physician will give you specific recommendations on your own individual renal diet. They will review factors such as your age, weight, blood test results, and your current urine output in preparing your diet.

Most likely, your renal diet will restrict your salt or sodium chloride intake to 2 grams a day. Sometimes food packages list their sodium content per serving in milligrams; 2 grams is equal to 2,000 milligrams. The need to restrict salt is due to salt retention caused by diseased kidneys. We excrete most of our salt in the urine and a small amount in sweat. If a dialysis patient eats too much salt, he or she may have high blood pressure. This can put a strain on the heart or lead to a stroke. If the heart becomes overloaded by too much salt and water, it may fail to pump enough blood, causing shortness of breath as fluid backs up into the lungs. Potassium is another salt that must be restricted to 2 grams, or 2,000 milligrams, a day. Potassium is inside all of the cells that make up our body. If the potassium level in the blood gets too high, it can cause heart problems and muscle weakness. A high potassium level can be diagnosed by a blood test or by an EKG of the heart. Some foods that are high in potassium include oranges, orange juice, cantaloupe, bananas, and tomatoes.

Phosphorus is an important mineral because it is needed to store energy from food for later use. It is also present in our bones. The only way we can excrete phosphorus from our body is through our kidneys. As our kidney function decreases, phosphorus builds up in our bloodstream, causing calcium in our blood to be deposited back into our bones. As the blood-calcium level falls, it stimulates the production of parathyroid hormone, called PTH for short, by the parathyroid gland. Parathyroid hormone will cause more calcium to be absorbed in our small intestine. It will also cause the release of too much calcium from our bones, which can lead to weakening of our bones and even fractures. We must control the phosphorus level in our blood to keep our bones healthy. This is accomplished by taking medications called phosphate binders that bind phosphorus that we eat in our intestine. We also must decrease the amount of phosphorus we eat every day. Phosphorus is contained in meat, dairy products, and beans, such as lentils and kidney beans.

Protein is an important part of the renal diet. You need to eat about 1.2 grams of protein per kilogram of body weight, which is 7 to 8 ounces of meat, chicken, or fish a day. Many people are under the impression that they should not eat protein if they are a kidney dialysis patient. This advice is wrong and could lead to protein malnutrition. Protein is needed to build and repair muscles, make blood cells, fight infection, and perform many other metabolic tasks in our body.

How many calories are needed every day? This depends on our age, how physically active we are, and how much we weigh. About 30 kilocalories per kilogram, or 2,000 to 2,500 calories, will be the ideal daily range for most kidney dialysis patients.

Your own personal diet will also depend on other medical problems. If you have an elevated cholesterol level or diabetes, these conditions will be taken into account when your dietitian and physician formulate your renal diet. Most patients begin to learn about their diet on the first day of dialysis. The dietitian often introduces himself or herself and gives the patient a diet sheet. He or she will remind the patient that alternatives to the diet sheet are possible and will review favorite foods that can fit into the renal diet. The patient then meets the social worker, doctor, and nurses in the dialysis unit. Then they have their first treatment. When patients first look at the diet sheet, they focus on their favorite foods that are prohibited, increasing their feeling of loss. Not only will they be stuck on dialysis, but they will never be able to eat normal foods again. I prefer to think of the renal diet as a voyage. We start in one place and slowly travel to another place. Many patients have some residual renal function when they start dialysis. This means that they are making urine and getting rid of some toxins and poisons, but not enough to stay off dialysis. The renal diet is not as important at the beginning of dialysis as it will be later on when the residual renal function is gone. Most patients have time to adjust to the renal diet. At the beginning of your dialysis treatments, you should concentrate on one or two important points. This may be to decrease your fluid and salt intake. You may be already accustomed to eating a low-salt diet. Ask your doctor and dietitian to tell you the most important part of the renal diet for you. This will prevent you from being overwhelmed and help you concentrate on getting used to your dialysis treatments. Later on, you can learn more when you are feeling better physically and psychologically. Your ability to manage your diet will improve. You will head in the right direction and develop healthier eating habits. Remember that all worthwhile voyages take time.

Erick Lucero writes:

My wife does the cooking in our family. She eats the same food as I do. She doesn't mind the renal diet, and we both try to eat healthy. We have a pamphlet prepared by a nutritionist, which is like a menu. It plans meals on the renal diet for several days. We eat a lot of chicken. I eat a small amount of tomatoes once a week. Instead of oranges, I try to eat lots of raspberries and blueberries. I am a Mexican-American, and a lot of our traditional foods are not on the renal diet. Once in a while, I eat some beans with hot sauce. I watch my lab tests to make sure my potassium and phosphorus levels are not high because of my diet. My father died young at age 51. I want to take good care of myself because I have a young daughter to take care of. I want to live as long a life as I can.

59. Can I eat more foods on peritoneal dialysis?

Yes, one of the joys of peritoneal dialysis is the ability to eat more varieties of food. Patients on hemodialysis must restrict their diet to about 1 to 1½ quarts or liters of fluid a day. Hemodialysis is an intermittent therapy. This means that you are receiving a treatment and then fluid and poisons will build up in your body for 2 days before you will have another treatment. In peritoneal dialysis, you are receiving treatment throughout the day every day. Fluid is removed every day. Potassium is usually a little low or normal, allowing you to eat orange juice, potatoes, tomatoes, and other high-potassium foods. Phosphorus, which is restricted on hemodialysis, is also removed on a daily basis on peritoneal dialysis. Patients on peritoneal dialysis can eat more dairy products such as milk, ice cream, and cheese. Beans and meats also contain phosphorus.

One would think that everyone would want to be on peritoneal dialysis so they could avoid a restrictive renal diet. However, peritoneal dialysis is less efficient than hemodialysis. This means that very large patients are not able to remove enough toxins and poisons to prevent the complications of renal failure. Patients who do well on peritoneal dialysis have some residual renal function. Their kidneys still produce some urine and this helps eliminate more poisons. It is also important to determine if you are willing to be on dialysis every day. As a peritoneal dialysis patient, you will be doing your own dialysis. This allows flexibility but also requires responsibility. If you think peritoneal dialysis may be for you, talk to your dialysis team. They can put you in contact with a peritoneal dialysis nurse. This nurse has a great deal of experience in treating patients on peritoneal dialysis. He or she can give you specific scientific information about peritoneal dialysis and introduce you to patients on peritoneal dialysis. You will be able to hear in these patients' own words the advantages of being on peritoneal dialysis.

It is important to mention that daily nocturnal home dialysis also allows the patient to eat and drink a larger variety of foods. This is because dialysis is typically done 6 or 7 days a week. Fluid, salt, potassium,

As a peritoneal dialysis patient, you will be doing your own dialysis. This allows flexibility but also requires responsibility.

phosphorus, toxins, and poisons are all removed on a daily basis. This allows you to eat at your favorite restaurant, then go home and remove all of the substances that can cause problems just like your own kidneys would. Make sure you consider daily nocturnal dialysis if you like to eat.

Patients with renal failure who choose to have a kidney transplant have an increased variety of food choices. Many transplant patients must still restrict the amount of salt they eat because they may still tend to retain salt. They can drink more fluid and eat more potassium and phosphorus than hemodialysis patients. They must still pay attention to their cholesterol intake if they have a high cholesterol level. Diabetic patients will still be diabetic when they are on renal replacement therapy. Many diabetic patients will have a better appetite when they begin dialysis, resulting in an increased intake of calories and an increased blood sugar. It is important to realize that you will need to adjust your diabetes medications after you start renal replacement therapy.

60. How much fluid should I drink every day?

The amount of fluid that you can safely drink on dialysis will depend on the amount of urine you make. If you continue to make a large amount of urine, you are very lucky. This will allow you to drink more. Before you begin dialysis, your doctor will probably order a 24-hour urine collection for creatinine clearance. This important test will determine if you need to start dialysis. It will also give you an idea of how much urine you are producing every day. Most of us have no idea.

We know how many times we urinate but not how much. If you are making a quart of urine a day, you can add that amount to the 1 to 1½ quarts of fluid you should drink each day. If you think in liters and kilograms, that is okay too. Some dialysis units use pounds of weight, but most use kilograms when they weigh you before and after dialysis.

On a daily basis, it is too much work to measure every fluid you drink. You may want to perform this useful exercise once or twice, but life is too short to measure every drop that goes into your body. Fortunately, if you gain 1 kilogram of weight, that corresponds to 1 liter of fluid that you drank. This formula enables us to determine if you are drinking too much. If you drink 1 liter of fluid and urinate 1 liter of fluid, you will lose weight. This seeming imbalance is due to **insensible fluid loss**. Insensible fluid loss is fluid lost in our bowel movements in the form of stool, in sweat, and through water vapor from our lungs. Insensible loss is about one-half to three-quarters of a liter of fluid a day. So, we measure our urine output, add one-half a liter a day of insensible loss of fluid, and another liter a day of fluid that is to be removed on dialysis, and we get a figure that is roughly 1½ to 2 liters of fluid a day. Do not worry if you are confused. Just weigh yourself after dialysis and plan to gain 2 kilograms or 4.4 pounds before your next treatment. Either method will work.

Many patients on dialysis are very thirsty. The exact reason for this is not known. It may be due to the effect of hormones released by the body, or it may be a signal from the brain that causes patients to seek water to drink. Some medications for blood pressure such as clonidine can make your mouth dry. Many patients resort to eating ice to decrease their thirst.

Insensible fluid loss

The fluid that leaves the body in the form of water vapor from the lungs, sweat, and fluid in stool. The amount of insensible fluid loss is about 2 to 3 cups every day.

Unfortunately, melted ice is water, and this is not an ideal solution. It is important to have some sugar-free gum or candy to pop in your mouth when you become thirsty. This will decrease the amount of fluid you consume. It is also important to have a sense of the fluid content of foods. The best example would be watermelon, which contains a large amount of fluid.

61. Can I eat protein on dialysis?

Many people believe that eating protein is harmful to the kidney and may be unhealthy for patients on dialysis. The nutritional content of the food we eat can be divided into protein, carbohydrate, and fat. In the early days of treatment for kidney failure, there was no dialysis. Physicians discovered that reducing the protein intake of patients allowed them to live longer because they produced less poisons and toxins on a low-protein diet. Patients became malnourished but had less symptoms of kidney failure. In the 1980s, a series of experiments with rats showed that rats with kidney failure lived longer on a low-protein rat chow diet than rats with kidney failure on a regular-protein rat chow diet. This research rekindled the interest in low-protein diets in kidney failure. Studies in humans failed to show a clear benefit of low-protein diet in patients with kidney failure. The only role for reducing protein in the diet may be in the pre-dialysis period. Some physicians feel that placing patients on a 30- to 40-gram protein diet may help keep them off dialysis for a time.

The danger of decreasing protein in the diet is the development of protein malnutrition. Protein in the food we eat is broken down into smaller building blocks called **amino acids**. These amino acids are used

Amino acids

Organic acids that are the building blocks of proteins.

to make blood cells, repair injured or damaged organs, make messenger proteins in our blood, and build muscle. If our protein intake and calories are too low, our body begins to use the protein in our own muscle as a fuel source, which leads to **muscle wasting**. This condition can result in weakness, fatigue, anemia, and a decreased ability to repair our body when injured. It can also lead to a decreased ability to fight infection. Anyone considering a low-protein diet for kidney failure should be observed carefully for malnutrition. This is especially important in children, elderly patients, and patients who are losing large amounts of protein in the urine.

Most doctors and nutritionists recommend that patients with kidney failure eat a good amount of **high-biologic-value protein** each day. What is high-biologic-value protein? High-biologic-value protein is protein that contains all of the essential amino acids that we need and that can be easily absorbed by our digestive system. Some amino acids can be built by our body. Essential amino acids cannot be built by the body and must be eaten and absorbed. Many vegetables contain protein, but they do not contain all of the essential amino acids needed for good nutrition. Patients who are vegetarians must take special care to eat a variety of foods that will provide them with all of their protein requirements. This means eating 1.2 grams of protein per kilogram of body weight. This nutritional requirement can be satisfied by eating 4 ounces of meat, poultry, or fish twice a day. Most of us have no idea of the weight in grams or ounces of the food we eat. Your renal dietitian can help you determine the portion size of food that is needed for good nutrition. Food models are available to help you understand portion size.

Muscle wasting

A decrease in the size of the muscles of the body due to poor nutrition or medical illness.

High-biologic-value protein

Proteins found in foods such as eggs, fish, poultry, soy products, and meat. High-biologic-value proteins are easily digestible and are rich in the ten essential amino acids that our body cannot make.

If you are not eating enough protein, you can use protein supplements, which are available in a powder or liquid form. Supplements can be especially helpful if your appetite is poor and if your protein stores have been depleted by illness. Many patients have a poor appetite in the pre-dialysis period because poisons and toxins are building up in their body, and they lose interest in their favorite foods. It is interesting that some patients selectively decrease the amount of protein they eat. These patients may be trying to decrease the amount of poisons and toxins they produce. Patients in the pre-dialysis period often lose weight and some of their protein stores. They may suffer from nausea, vomiting, and hiccups, which interfere with eating. These symptoms usually resolve within several weeks of dialysis treatments. Infections occurring in patients on dialysis can lead to protein malnutrition. Examples of this would be foot infections, access infections, or pneumonia. Attention to adequate nutrition during these episodes of infection can help speed recovery and return you to your normal routine.

62. Can I eat during my dialysis treatments?

If you are a peritoneal dialysis patient, you will be eating during your dialysis treatments. Dialysis is taking place 24 hours a day. The dialysis usually does not interfere with the ability to eat an adequate diet. Peritoneal dialysate contains a sugar called **dextrose** that helps remove fluid from the bloodstream into the peritoneal space so it can be discarded with the dialysate. Some dextrose is absorbed by the body. These extra calories from the dextrose can sometimes act as an appetite suppressor and decrease the patient's desire to

Dextrose

A sugar added to peritoneal dialysis solutions to help remove fluid from the body. It is also added to intravenous fluids to provide calories for nutrition.

eat. Occasionally, patients feel full when their abdomen is full of dialysate. This symptom can be managed by having the patient eat when the abdomen is drained of dialysate.

Hemodialysis centers have different policies regarding patients eating on hemodialysis. You definitely should not eat during hemodialysis in the first few weeks of your treatment. Many patients have episodes of vomiting as the high levels of poisons and toxins are removed during their first hemodialysis treatment. You definitely do not want to have a full stomach. After adjusting to hemodialysis, many patients find that eating a small snack during their treatment is enjoyable. This may be especially important in patients who are diabetic and who are regulating their glucose. It is important to talk to your dialysis nursing staff to find out the eating policy in your hemodialysis unit. Patients on home hemodialysis frequently combine dialysis with their dinner plans. They come home from work, receive their dialysis treatment, and enjoy having dinner with their family while they are receiving their treatment. This can help with a busy schedule and create time for other activities.

After adjusting to hemodialysis, many patients find that eating a small snack during their treatment is enjoyable.

63. Why are potassium and phosphorus so important?

If you spend time in any dialysis unit, you will hear the patients, nurses, dieticians, and doctors talking about these two important elements. Potassium and phosphorus occur inside and outside the cells in our body. They are both needed for healthy living. Potassium and phosphorus levels in our blood reflect the quality of the dialysis treatment and how successful we are in following the renal diet.

Most of the potassium is inside the cells in our body. It also is present in a smaller amount in the liquid part of our blood or serum. Potassium is eaten in our food every day and excreted in our urine, stool, and sweat. In patients with kidney failure, the ability to eliminate potassium in the urine decreases. In order to compensate, we must decrease our intake of potassium in our food and increase our elimination of potassium with the help of the dialysis treatment. We cannot measure the potassium inside the cells of our body. We use the potassium level in our blood to determine if the potassium in our body is at an optimal level. A potassium level that is too high or too low can cause panic in the dialysis unit. This reaction is because very high and very low levels can be associated with heart problems. Irregular or slow heartbeats and cardiac standstill, called cardiac arrest, have been associated with these extreme potassium levels. Muscle weakness and even paralysis are other signs of an abnormally high potassium level. Most patients with these levels do not develop these problems, but it is important to correct a low or high potassium level as soon as possible.

The most common cause of a high potassium level is eating too much potassium in the diet. Orange juice, bananas, cantaloupe, dairy products, tomatoes, salt substitutes, and sports drinks such as Gatorade have too much potassium in them to be safe foods for the hemodialysis patient. The next common cause of a high potassium level is skipping dialysis treatments. An elevated potassium can also be due to a problem with the dialysis treatment. If the access that supplies blood to the hemodialysis machine is not working properly, not enough blood will pass over the dialysis membrane, and a decreased removal of potassium occurs. If there is a blockage in the access, the same blood can go from the patient to the machine over and over again without mixing with the rest of the blood in the body. This is called **recirculation** and is prevented by a frequent evaluation of the a-v access. Patients can also liberate too much potassium from the organs in their body due to disease. This can occur during crush injuries when damaged muscle lets large amounts of potassium that is usually found inside the cells to leak out into the bloodstream. Another cause of a high potassium level is bleeding in the gastrointestinal tract from an ulcer or an inflammation of the lining of the stomach, known as gastritis. Red blood cells contain large amounts of potassium, which can be absorbed from the bowel.

The immediate treatment of a high potassium level in a dialysis patient should be to place the patient on dialysis as soon as possible. At the same time, an evaluation should be made of the cause of the high potassium and steps should be taken to decrease the potassium intake in the diet. Low potassium can be the result of vomiting and diarrhea, laxative use, or a decrease in appetite leading to a very low intake of potassium over a long period of time. This problem can often be managed by changing the potassium level in the dialysate and improving the patient's nutritional intake.

Phosphorus, like potassium, is in the food we eat and is eliminated from the body in our urine. As our kidney function decreases, the level of phosphorus in the blood begins to rise. This is managed by decreasing the

Recirculation

Occurs during hemodialysis treatments when blood that has gone through the dialysis machine does not mix with the patient's blood but returns to the dialysis machine.

amount of phosphorus we eat. High phosphorus foods include meat, dairy products, beans, and cola drinks. In addition to eating a reduced phosphorus diet, most dialysis patients will require phosphate binders. These medicines are taken with food and will bind the phosphorus in the gastrointestinal tract and prevent the phosphorus from being absorbed. If the phosphorus level is too high, patients can complain of severe itching. In addition, the high phosphorus will cause the calcium in the blood to be deposited in the bones, causing the calcium level to fall, which will stimulate the production of parathyroid hormone (often referred to as PTH). The parathyroid hormone, if present in high levels, can cause bone disease that can cause pain or even fractures. Although a high phosphorus level is not as dangerous as a high potassium level, longstanding high phosphorus can affect the quality of a patient's life on dialysis and should be avoided. Low phosphorus is uncommon in dialysis patients. If your phosphorus is low, the first thing to do is decrease or stop your phosphorus binders. A small increase in the phosphorus in your diet may also be needed.

64. Can I smoke on dialysis?

A significant number of patients who smoke before they begin dialysis continue to smoke after they begin dialysis. All hemodialysis centers prohibit smoking while on dialysis. Many patients are surprised to learn that smoking cigarettes is an independent risk factor for kidney disease. This risk is because cigarette smoking is one of the causes of hardening of the arteries, or atherosclerosis. Atherosclerosis occurs all over the body. When it occurs in the arteries to the heart, heart disease or a heart attack occurs. Involvement of the

Because kidney patients have a higher chance of having hypertension and high cholesterol, it is especially important that they try to stop smoking.

arteries to the brain can lead to stroke. Atherosclerosis occuring in the arteries to the kidneys, results in a decreased blood supply to the kidney. Atherosclerosis is also caused by hypertension, diabetes, and high cholesterol, and occurs more frequently in patients who have other family members with the disease. Because kidney patients have a higher chance of having hypertension and high cholesterol, it is especially important that they try to stop smoking. Diabetic patients on hemodialysis are especially vulnerable to the effects of cigarette smoking. There is a significant decrease in 5-year survival in hemodialysis patients with diabetes who smoke.

Most smokers want to quit smoking and every year about half of them try to quit. Within 2 days of stopping, the ability to smell and taste food improves. Within 2 to 3 weeks, the chance of a heart attack decreases, and circulation and breathing begin to improve. It is important to obtain help from your doctor or a smoking cessation program. Their help will increase your chance of stopping smoking.

The first step in quitting smoking is to set a quit date in the coming weeks. During this time, you should write down your reasons for quitting smoking. You should also review behaviors that encourage you to smoke, such as drinking alcohol or being around other smokers, and try to avoid them. Contact your doctor about your plan to stop smoking. Ask him or her if nicotine replacement products or other medications might be helpful for you. Nicotine replacement therapy comes in transdermal patches, nicotine gum, lozenges, vapor inhalers, and nasal sprays. Other non-nicotine medications include bupropion, which is also known as Zyban and Wellbutrin. This medicine can be used with nicotine replacement. Varenicline, or Chantix, cannot be used with nicotine replacement therapy and has to be used with great caution in patients with kidney failure at a reduced dose. Get rid of ash trays, cigarettes, and other objects that are associated with smoking. Make your home into a smoke-free zone. If other family members smoke, ask them not to smoke in front of you. Tell your friends and family of your plans to quit, and get their support. Withdrawal from smoking peaks within 1 to 3 weeks after quitting. Be prepared for withdrawal symptoms such as depression, craving for cigarettes, and difficulty concentrating. Beginning dialysis may be the ideal time to consider quitting smoking. You will be getting a great deal of attention from the dialysis team. You will be focused on learning healthy lifestyle choices and may be more motivated than when you get more accustomed to your dialysis treatments.

65. How can I improve my appetite?

Kidney patients on dialysis have many reasons for having a poor appetite. Poisons and toxins that build up in the body of a patient with kidney failure change the way food tastes and smells. It is interesting that smell is such an important sense in good nutrition. If we cannot smell a food or if the smell of a food is not pleasing, we will reject that food. Many patients report a metallic taste in their mouth, which is due to poisons and toxins that are building up in the body. Kidney patients may have a dry mouth, which may cause them to drink large amounts of fluid with no nutritional value, leaving them too full to eat solid foods with more nutrition. Nausea, vomiting, and hiccups are common symptoms of kidney failure in the pre-dialysis period. Patients become afraid that eating will cause them to vomit.

Beginning dialysis will reverse some, but not all of these symptoms. Many patients who delay beginning dialysis will spend several months with poor nutritional intake. As they lose weight, they become physically weaker and less mobile. They suffer from nausea, a decreased appetite, and general malaise. These symptoms decrease their interest in and ability to consume an adequate amount of food. They become accustomed to eating less. When they begin dialysis, they have to get in the habit of eating more again. Patients are often overwhelmed by the renal diet that is presented to them. They may be unsure of what is safe for them to eat. All patients who begin dialysis have an element of depression present. Patients often feel that beginning dialysis is a loss and that life as they knew it is over. This depression is often associated with a decreased appetite.

Improving your appetite and nutrition is fortunately not as hard as it seems. The first thing is to realize that your diet is equally as important as your dialysis treatments and medication in getting well.

Improving your appetite and nutrition is fortunately not as hard as it seems. The first thing is to realize that your diet is equally as important as your dialysis treatments and medication in getting well. Eating is a social experience. We celebrate special occasions like birthdays and holidays with a special meal. You will eat more if you share your meals with family and friends. If you are in the hospital, have a friend or family member visit you at mealtimes. Have them bring a sandwich so they can eat with you. This will help distract you from eating as a task to get through and reconnect you with food as a pleasurable experience. Eat five small meals or snacks a day. Patients who fill up on small amounts of food can let their stomachs empty a bit before they eat again. If you need to consume more calories, do not eat or drink anything with the word diet or low-fat in it. I am always amazed to find patients who are in very poor nutritional health eating a low-fat yogurt or diet soda. What is a good idea for well-nourished individuals may not be the best food for malnourished people. Make sure that everything that goes into you has some caloric value. If you are thirsty, drink a liquid supplement or apple juice, not water. Avoid carbonated beverages. The bubbles can distend your stomach and make you feel full, leaving less room for food. It is important to remember that just about everyone who stops smoking gains a few pounds. If you smoke, this may be the perfect time to quit and gain weight.

Physical activity is one of the best ways to increase your appetite. Active people consume a great deal of calories. They are less likely to suffer from constipation and other bowel complaints. Try to take a short walk several times a day. Find a reason to go out even if you do not have to. Buy a newspaper or pick up a quart of milk or juice. Resist the urge to sit and watch television. Do some work around the house or the garden, even if it is only a small task that can easily be done by someone else. All these activities will increase your appetite.

Medications are sometimes used to increase appetite. Megace is a synthetic derivative of the naturally occurring hormone progesterone. It has been used to treat patients with anorexia and severe malnutrition with wasting, called cachexia. We do not know why Megace works, but it can stimulate appetite and food intake in some patients with kidney failure. It is available as a liquid and must be prescribed by your physician. Another medication that can sometimes be helpful is zinc supplements. Zinc is a metal. Patients with zinc deficiency can lose their taste for foods. Antidepressants can help some depressed patients with kidney failure gain weight. These drugs are called serotonin reuptake inhibitors, or SRIs for short, and must be prescribed by physicians who are expert in their use. Although medications are usually not an easy answer to the problem of poor appetite, they may be useful in selected patients.

66. Who will help me improve my nutrition?

Every dialysis unit has a key person who will be available to help you with your nutrition. This person is the renal dietitian. He or she will have special scientific training to help you understand your nutritional condition, choose healthy nutritious food, and act as your nutritional advocate. It is sad for me to say that I had 1 or 2 days of my medical school curriculum devoted to nutrition. During my training in internal medicine and nephrology, I learned to diagnose nutritional problems but received very little training on the treatment of nutritional disorders. I need to work closely with the dietitian in my dialysis unit, who is a major resource and guide in all matters related to food and nutritional supplements. Dietitians are helpful people. They want to understand where you are coming from. All of us have particular likes and dislikes when it comes to food. The magic of the dietitian is the ability to help you choose food that tastes good and that is good for you. Patients on dialysis come from many different cultures and backgrounds. They are used to eating ethnic foods that may or may not be appropriate for patients with kidney failure. Often the renal dietitian can recommend substitutions in the recipe of your favorite food to make the food more compatible with the renal diet.

The tools that the renal dietitian will use to evaluate your nutritional state are the monthly blood tests that you will be taking and your height and weight. One of the most important values will be the serum **albumin**. This blood test is a reflection of the protein stores in your body. The albumin level can be low for a variety of reasons. You may be malnourished and not eating enough protein. You may be losing albumin in your urine because of your kidney disease. You may be suffering from liver disease and may not be able to build enough albumin protein despite adequate protein intake. The other important lab values include your BUN and creatinine, your phosphorus and calcium levels, and your cholesterol level. If your cholesterol level is too low, it may be a sign that you are not eating enough food. The renal dietitian can use these tests along with your height and weight to give you a nutritional snapshot of where you are now. The more you understand, the better you will be at improving your nutritional condition. Good nutrition will allow you to build muscle and become stronger. It will give you more energy to participate in important events such as family gatherings and will help you return to work if this is your goal.

Most of us are not used to getting advice about our diet. It is important for you to realize that the advice of the renal dietitian is not an attack on your food choices. It is rather an observation on how your food choices will affect your health in the long run. You should always ask your dietitian which dietary recommendation is the most important. This will help you

Albumin

A water-soluble protein found in the blood normally in very minute amounts. Patients with kidney disease often have albumin in their urine because the albumin leaks through the damaged kidneys into the urine.

concentrate on the one change that will help you the most. Remember, the renal diet is a voyage. You are in one place, and you are hoping to arrive at another place, which is healthier. It will take longer than you think to accomplish your goals. Think of the renal dietitian as a fellow traveler. Explain why you feel the way you do about the particular route he or she has suggested. Remember that the renal dietitian has taken this voyage innumerable times following many different paths. With his or her help, try to find the right path for you.

Gastroenterologist

A physician who has received training in internal medicine and who has had additional training in the diagnosis and treatment of disorders of the digestive system.

Many other people will be available to help your nutrition, including your physician and nurses in the unit. Some patients with specific medical diseases may have a **gastroenterologist**. Many gastroenterologists have special training in nutrition. The American Association of Kidney Patients, *www.aakp.org*, has a wonderful publication called *Beginnings, Living Well With Kidney Disease*. This publication features many excellent articles concerning nutrition and recipes for great meals, and it is an enjoyable resource for patients on kidney dialysis. Other great recipes can be found at *www.culinary kidneycooks.com* and *www.kidney-cookbook.com*.

PART SIX

Complications on Dialysis

What should I do if I develop bleeding from my access?

Why does my blood pressure fall too low during my hemodialysis treatment?

Why do I feel weak after my hemodialysis treatments?

More ...

67. Why is my access so important?

You will be hearing a great deal about access even before you begin your dialysis treatments. The word access includes a variety of devices all used to gain access to the blood circulation. In hemodialysis, the best access is a fistula. The fistula is a tube created by a surgeon in the operating room, by connecting an artery to a vein in the arm (**Figure 7**). Blood from the artery causes the vein in the arm to enlarge and for the wall of the vein to become thicker. The fistula will take 6 weeks to 3 months or more to be ready for use. When it is ready, two needles are inserted into the fistula. One needle will be connected to plastic tubing that will bring blood to the dialysis machine. After the blood has been cleaned of poisons and toxins, the blood will travel through plastic tubing and be returned through a second needle. The fistula is the access of choice for hemodialysis because it will last the longest, be resistant to infection, and be able to repair itself if damaged because it is constructed of living artery and vein.

The fistula is most commonly inserted in the lower arm. It can also be placed in the upper arm and, very rarely, in the patient's upper leg. The fistula takes time to develop or mature. This maturation process can sometimes be facilitated by inserting a small, long balloon in the fistula and inflating the balloon. This process, called **angioplasty**, can increase the size of the vein and enable it to have more blood flowing through the fistula. Angioplasty can help make the fistula ready to use earlier and will make the dialysis more effective because more blood will go through the dialysis machine during a given time.

Angioplasty

A medical procedure in which a balloon catheter is inserted into a blood vessel or dialysis access. When the balloon is inflated, it opens a blockage in the blood vessel to improve blood flow.

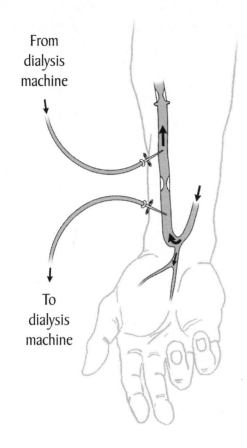

From
dialysis
machine

To
dialysis
machine

Figure 7   An A-V fistula

Source: National Institute of Diabetes and Digestive and Kidney Diseases, National Institutes of Health.

Over time, the fistula can have too much blood flow and decrease the amount of blood to the hand, making the hand painful, cold, and pale. This is called a **steal syndrome** because the fistula steals blood from the hand. The cold, painful, pale hand is said to be **ischemic**. This term describes the lack of blood flow to the hand. If steal syndrome occurs, surgery may be required to place a band around the fistula, reducing blood flow through the fistula so more blood can go to the hand. If the ischemia is severe, the fistula may need

Steal syndrome

A syndrome that occurs when too much blood is taken away from the arm or hand by an a-v fistula or a-v graft. The blood goes from the artery to the vein, bypassing the capillaries to the hand or arm, resulting in coolness, pain, and sometimes loss of function of the hand.

Ischemia

A decrease or lack of blood flow to an organ in the body causing damage or organ dysfunction.

to be closed off to reestablish blood flow to the hand. This is done by having a vascular surgeon place a suture, which is a sterile piece of plastic string, around the fistula and tie a tight knot. The suture causes the blood to stop flowing and the fistula to stop working.

Another complication of fistulas is aneurysm formation. The aneurysm is an outpouching of the vein part of the fistula. This looks like a small balloon and can rupture and cause bleeding if it gets very large. Aneurysms of the fistula must be observed carefully by the vascular surgeon and fixed before they rupture. A fistula can develop a blockage. If this happens, you should immediately contact your doctor to have it fixed as soon as possible. The blockage is sometimes caused by scarring of a portion of the vein and that decreases the blood flow through the fistula and causes the blood to clot. The clot can be removed during a procedure called **thrombectomy**, and a small amount of dye can be injected into the fistula to diagnose the cause of the blockage. If there is a narrowing of the vein, it can be fixed by using a balloon to do an angioplasty to increase the blood flow through the fistula. The fistula should be protected at all times. Blood should not be drawn from the arm with the fistula to prevent damage to the fistula. Tight-fitting jewelry and clothing should never constrict the fistula because this may cause it to clot. Blood pressure should never be taken on the arm with the fistula.

Thrombectomy

A procedure in which a blood clot that is blocking a blood vessel or an a-v access is removed or dissolved with medication. It allows blood to flow through the hemodialysis access so it can be used for hemodialysis.

If the veins in the arms are not very large, an arterial-venous graft, or a-v graft, can be the next best choice for access (**Figure 8**). The graft is constructed by sewing a plastic tube between an artery and a vein. The plastic tube is composed of a material called Gortex. This tube is tunneled under the skin. After about 2 to 3

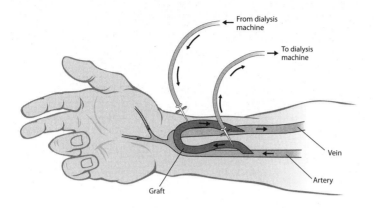

From dialysis machine

To dialysis machine

Vein

Artery

Graft

Figure 8 An A-V graft

Source: National Institute of Diabetes and Digestive and Kidney Diseases, National Institutes of Health.

weeks, the swelling after surgery will decrease and the graft will be ready for use. At the beginning of the hemodialysis treatment, two needles are inserted into the plastic tube. Arterial-venous grafts have a high rate of clotting (or thrombosis) and generally last about 9 months to 3 years, making them a poor choice for patients who will need to be treated with hemodialysis for many years. This access will wear out after repeated needle insertions. If the a-v graft gets infected, it will need to be surgically removed because the infection will never really go away. Grafts also can develop blockages and aneurysms, which can be surgically repaired.

The third type of access for hemodialysis is the dialysis catheter (**Figure 9**). The dialysis catheter is a piece of plastic tubing that is inserted in a vein in the neck or leg. A catheter can be temporary, and used for one or two dialysis treatments, or more permanent and used for weeks to months. Catheters can be used right away, as soon as they are inserted. Needles are not necessary so there is no pain associated with using the catheter

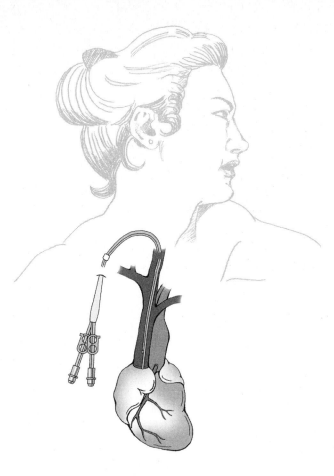

Figure 9   A hemodialysis catheter

Source: National Institute of Diabetes and Digestive and Kidney Diseases, National Institutes of Health.

for hemodialysis. Catheters are not good accesses for several reasons. The catheter exits the skin and is sutured and taped to the patient's body. This allows bacteria from the skin to enter the bloodstream and cause serious infection. Catheters can also cause scarring of the vein, which can lead to a blockage of the vein and make it impossible to put a fistula in the arm closest to the catheter. Catheters become blocked, kinked, and wear out. You should not get your catheter wet. This means no bathing, showers, or swimming. You must use sponge baths to keep the catheter from becoming infected. I think of a hemodialysis catheter as a temporary access. The next step after getting a catheter for hemodialysis is planning to have an a-v fistula made so the catheter can be removed as soon as possible.

The access in peritoneal dialysis is the peritoneal dialysis catheter. This access is a plastic tube that is inserted into the lower abdomen during a minor surgical procedure. The peritoneal dialysis catheter will take about 2 weeks to heal. This is so tissue can form a seal around the catheter so it does not leak fluid around the catheter. The peritoneal dialysis catheter is used to instill dialysate fluid into the peritoneum where it can draw poisons and toxins into the fluid. The fluid is then drained out by gravity, and fresh dialysate is then infused into the abdomen. Like hemodialysis catheters, peritoneal catheters can be blocked and infected. The catheter can work its way out of the abdomen and could need to be replaced. Your peritoneal dialysis nurse will teach you how to care for your access during your training. Keeping the access clean is called **exit site care** and is done every day. It involves washing the area where the catheter exits the skin in the abdomen with an antiseptic solution, called saline. The exit site is then covered with a sterile dressing. Special care is required not to put too much tension on the catheter and to secure it to the abdomen so it will not move with exercise. Exit site care is done after showering, swimming, or vigorous exercise. This is to decrease the chance of the catheter developing an irritation at the exit site that could lead to an infection.

Exit site care

Exit site care involves swabbing the area where the peritoneal dialysis catheter exits the skin with an antiseptic solution and covering the exit site with a clean sterile dressing.

68. What is an access center?

In the early days of dialysis, the access was inserted by surgeons in the operating room of the hospital. As medical science improved, new techniques were developed. Hemodialysis catheters were invented for temporary use. Fistulas created in the operating room that do not develop properly are enlarged with the use of a procedure called balloon angioplasty (Question 67). Fistulas and grafts that develop clots can have the clots dissolved. Many times the patient would have to wait several days for a simple access procedure because there was no time in the operating room of the hospital. Patients would have their procedure cancelled because of emergencies such as appendicitis or trauma cases. Because of the increasing number of dialysis patients, the **access center** was developed to care for dialysis patients with access-related complications.

Access center

A medical facility that specializes in the creation and care of access for dialysis patients. The access physician uses radiology and ultrasound equipment to evaluate and improve the blood flow in a-v fistulas, a-v grafts, and catheters for hemodialysis.

The access center is often not a part of the hospital. The access center has a physician with special training in dialysis access. The physician could be a surgeon, nephrologist, or radiologist. This physician only works on dialysis access, enabling him or her to develop advanced skills and techniques through specialization and focusing on one problem. The access physician understands the importance of fixing the access as soon as possible. The access physician will have nurses and technicians with special training in access procedures as assistants. Access centers are set up to provide superior care as rapidly as possible. Access centers often allow patients to have their access fixed and to return to the hemodialysis unit the same day for their treatment. They can prevent the need for admission to the hospital and often avoid extra procedures such as the insertion of temporary dialysis catheters. If a dialysis catheter is needed, the access center can insert it. If it is time to remove your catheter because your a-v fistula is working well and your catheter is no longer needed, they can remove it. The access center is often a more pleasant environment than the hospital operating room. Patients in the access center are all on dialysis and are not as sick as patients in holding areas of the operating room of a hospital. The staff is trained about the special needs of dialysis patients and will get to know you and your nephrologist. This will help you get the access care you need with minimal complications and disruption of your dialysis schedule.

Access centers are set up to provide superior care as rapidly as possible.

69. What should I do if I develop bleeding from my access?

Bleeding from the a-v fistula or a-v graft is one of the most common complications of hemodialysis. Bleeding is very upsetting to the patient and dialysis staff, but most of the time it is not life threatening. The first thing to do if you develop bleeding is to apply direct pressure to the part of the access that is bleeding. This can be done with sterile gauze. If you are not in the dialysis unit and do not have a sterile gauze, a clean handkerchief, paper towel, or any clean cloth can be used. If there is a great deal of blood loss, the best thing to do is call 911 and have the emergency medical technician come to your home. This person will take your blood pressure and pulse, put a clean pressure dressing on the access, and transport you to the emergency room for evaluation. If the bleeding is a small amount and stops with pressure, you may want to call or come to the dialysis unit if it is open for evaluation. Most of the time, bleeding occurs after your needles for hemodialysis are removed. This is because you have been given a blood thinner called heparin for your dialysis treatment. In this case, the bleeding can be stopped by applying direct pressure to the access. The heparin will be metabolized by your body and the bleeding will stop.

Bleeding from your access on a day you are not on dialysis is a sure sign that something is wrong with the access.

Bleeding from your access on a day you are not on dialysis is a sure sign that something is wrong with the access. It may indicate that the access has an infection. In this case, the bleeding may be accompanied by redness and warmth of the access. Fever may also be present. Infection can be confirmed by obtaining blood cultures to find the bacteria in the blood. A surgeon may have to perform a small incision in the skin to evaluate the problem. During the procedure, if the surgeon sees pus, which is caused by white blood cells attacking the bacteria, he or she may take cultures and have to remove the access if it is an a-v graft. The surgeon may try to remove the infected part of the graft, but this can often fail to control the infection. It is important that medical evaluation is not delayed. A small amount of bleeding can be followed by rupture of the infected access and massive bleeding.

Another cause of access bleeding can be a blockage (or stenosis) at the outflow (or venous side) of the access. This can cause high pressure in the access, making it more likely that bleeding will occur at the needle puncture sites. This problem is best treated by inserting a small balloon across the area with the blockage, inflating the balloon, and opening up the blockage. This procedure is called angioplasty. A surgeon can also fix the stenosis by making a small incision in the access and repairing it in the operating room. Bleeding can also occur from aneurysms of the a-v access. These weaknesses in the wall of the access can enlarge over time and be unsightly. When aneurysms bleed, this is a danger sign, and they should be evaluated by a vascular surgeon and repaired as soon as possible. As noted previously, many patients are on blood thinners that can promote bleeding from the access. Heparin is the most common medication given to prevent clotting while on hemodialysis. If you have frequent bleeding after your needles are removed, ask your nurse and doctor to consider decreasing your dose of heparin. Aspirin, Plavix, Persantine, and Coumadin are other medications that can contribute to bleeding from your access. If you have several episodes of bleeding from your access, your doctor may consider stopping these medications.

70. Why do I have anemia?

Anemia (low blood count) is a common complication of kidney failure. Symptoms of anemia include weakness, fatigue, and shortness of breath while exercising. You may feel your heart racing or beating fast with exertion. Your skin, nails, and lips may appear pale. One of the main reasons is that **red blood cells** have a shortened life span in kidney failure. Our red blood cells are made in our bone marrow from cells called stem cells. The cells are released into our circulation. In normal people, red blood cells last for 90 days in our circulation. Because kidney failure patients have poisons and toxins that remain in the blood despite dialysis, the red cells last much less than 90 days.

Our kidneys produce a hormone called erythropoietin. This protein is a messenger that tells the stem cells in the bone marrow to produce more red blood cells. Patients with kidney disease do not produce enough erythropoietin. Fortunately, erythropoietin is available

Red blood cells

Cells made by the bone marrow that contain an oxygen transport protein called hemoglobin, causing blood to appear red. Red blood cells carry oxygen from the lungs to other organs through the circulatory system.

as a medication that can be given by injecting it under the skin or intravenously. The brand names for erythropoietin are Epogen and Procrit. Another medication for anemia is called Aranesp. Many new medications for anemia are being developed.

Dialysis patients have frequent blood tests. They lose a little bit of blood that remains in the dialysis tubing at the end of the dialysis treatment. They may have blood loss because of bleeding in the gastrointestinal tract and have difficulty absorbing iron supplements from the gastrointestinal tract. Patients on dialysis often suffer from iron deficiency. Many dialysis units will replace iron deficiency by giving intravenous iron during the dialysis treatment. Chronic infection is another common cause of anemia. Chronic infection makes it difficult for the body to produce red blood cells even if erythropoietin and iron are given intravenously on hemodialysis. Good nutrition is important in maintaining a good blood cell count because red blood cells consist of hemoglobin, which is a protein that carries oxygen. Hemoglobin is composed of amino acids and iron. To build hemoglobin and red blood cells, a good intake of high-biologic-value protein is important.

Fortunately, blood transfusions are rarely required to treat anemia these days. Most hemodialysis patients will have their blood count checked every week. Iron stores are tested every month. Peritoneal dialysis patients have their blood tests every month. The successful treatment of anemia is one of the major goals of the dialysis team. You should discuss your blood count with your doctor and nurse when you review your monthly blood tests.

71. Why does my blood pressure fall too low during my hemodialysis treatment?

Your blood pressure will be measured at the beginning of your hemodialysis treatment and at frequent intervals during your treatment. When we remove fluid during hemodialysis treatments, the fluid removed comes directly from the blood within our circulation. Fluid that is present in cells and in other places will move into the circulation slowly. This lag in fluid entering the circulation can result in too little fluid being present in the arteries and veins of the circulatory system, making the blood pressure fall. Most dialysis patients have a decrease in blood pressure during their hemodialysis treatment because 3 to 4 liters of fluid are removed in a 3- to 4-hour treatment. Patients on peritoneal dialysis have a much slower continuous removal of fluid because they are on dialysis 24 hours a day, 7 days a week. This makes peritoneal dialysis a gentler, gradual dialysis treatment. One of the ways to prevent your blood pressure from falling during your hemodialysis treatment is to not drink an excessive amount of fluid between treatments. The more fluid removed, the more likely your blood pressure is to fall dramatically. Some patients find that taking their blood pressure medications after their dialysis treatment is useful. Ask your doctor if this is a good idea for you.

Low blood pressure is bad if you have symptoms. Symptoms of low blood pressure on hemodialysis include dizziness, palpitations or a racing heart beat, nausea, and vomiting or fainting. Many dialysis patients tolerate low blood pressure without symptoms. Occasionally patients begin their dialysis treatment

Complications on Dialysis

with low blood pressure and have a slight increase in blood pressure as their treatment progresses. The dialysis team will assess your blood pressure on a frequent basis and make changes in your dialysis treatment and medications to try to avoid low blood pressure.

72. My nurse told me my blood clotted in the hemodialysis machine during my treatment. Are these blood clots dangerous?

Our blood contains clotting factors that cause it to clot or turn from liquid into a solid at the right time. Clotting is beneficial when we injure or cut ourselves because the clot forms a plug to seal a hole in our blood vessels to stop bleeding. When blood comes out of our access, it comes into contact with steel needles, plastic tubing, and the dialysis membrane. All these devices tend to stimulate clot formation. Because of this tendency of blood to clot outside of the circulation, heparin, a blood thinner, is given at the beginning of the hemodialysis treatment. This medicine decreases, but does not eliminate, the chance that your blood will clot in the dialysis machine. If you have prolonged bleeding from your needle puncture sites after dialysis, your heparin dose may need to be decreased. If you have active bleeding in your gastrointestinal tract, your doctor may try to eliminate all heparin from your dialysis treatment. Another common cause of clot formation is low blood flow through the hemodialysis machine, which can occur if your dialysis needles are poorly positioned in your access. If the needle is touching the wall of your fistula or graft, it may be difficult to have a high dialysis blood flow. A blood count that is too high because a patient is receiving too much erythropoietin can also cause blood to clot.

One of the first signs of clot formation is an increase in pressure in the dialysis line. This can cause an alarm to go off and alert the nurse or dialysis technician of a problem. They will evaluate the cause of the increased pressure by flushing the tubing and dialyzer with saline solution, making it much easier to see a clot. If a clot progresses, you will be unable to continue your dialysis. If this happens, do not be alarmed. The clot cannot pass into your circulation and cause a medical problem. The nurse or technician will have to disconnect you from the dialysis machine, flush your needles with saline, and set up your machine with new tubing and a new dialyzer to continue your treatment. This occurrence is very common and will probably happen to you at some time if you are on hemodialysis. The blood lost by the tubing clotting is a small amount and is not dangerous. The worst thing that will happen is that your dialysis will take longer because the time it takes to replace your tubing and dialyzer should not be counted as time on dialysis. When you start dialysis, your dialysis team will start you on a heparin dose. They will increase the dose of heparin if you develop clots during your dialysis treatment, to help prevent you from forming more clots during your treatments.

73. Should I be concerned when the alarms go off on my hemodialysis machine?

The modern hemodialysis machine has many electronic sensors to alert the dialysis staff to a variety of events on dialysis. One alarm will sound when your

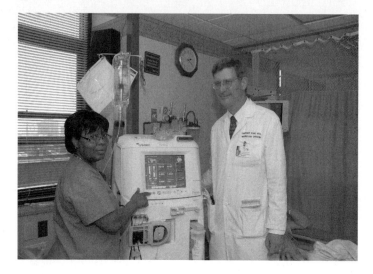

Figure 10   Frances Brebnor, RN, resets an alarm on a hemodiaysis machine.
Source: K. Neelakantappa, MD

treatment is finished, sort of like the alarm clock that wakes you from sleep. Other alarms will sound if the temperature of the blood or dialysate is too low or high. There are pressure sensors on the tubing bringing blood to the dialysis machine from your access and another pressure sensor for blood returning from the dialysis machine back to your access. The dialysis nurse can adjust these alarms (**Figure 10**). If blood leaks across the dialyzer into the dialysate, an alarm will sound. The most important sensor in the dialysis machine is the air bubble detector. The air bubble detector will shut down the blood pump and clamp the dialysis tubing to prevent the air from entering your access and traveling into your circulation. An alarm will sound to indicate the problem.

Safety sensors and alarms make dialysis safe. If you moved from the country to a busy city, you would be kept awake by the sounds of traffic, police, fire sirens, and car horns. It will take you some time to adjust to the sounds and lights of the sensors of your dialysis machine. You are not in danger when they sound. Most likely, nothing will immediately happen when they alarm. In several minutes, a dialysis team member will walk over to your hemodialysis machine, push a button or two, and then walk away as if nothing important has happened. Ask the staff member the meaning of the alarm. Many dialysis patients understand their dialysis machines and can figure out the meaning of the alarm on their own. Learning the meaning of hemodialysis machine alarms and what to do about them is a good exercise if you are considering going on home hemodialysis. At home, you and your dialysis partner will learn how to react to the alarms during your hemodialysis training. Patients on nocturnal home hemodialysis are asleep during their hemodialysis treatments. Because the blood flow on nocturnal dialysis is lower, there is less chance of an alarm going off during the hemodialysis treatment. A technician is awake monitoring many patients' machines at a remote location at the dialysis center. Nocturnal hemodialysis patients are monitored using the Internet. When an alarm goes off, the technician will call the patient to make sure he or she has correctly responded to the alarm.

Safety sensors and alarms make dialysis safe. You are not in danger when they sound.

The peritoneal dialysis machine is also known as a cycler. It will instill dialysate into the abdomen, drain the dialysate, and repeat the process. Peritoneal dialysis machines are often used at night while the patient sleeps. The most common cause of an alarm on peritoneal dialysis is bent or kinked tubing preventing dialysate flow. The alarm will alert the patient that a problem has occurred but does not indicate a dangerous situation.

74. Why do I feel weak after my hemodialysis treatments?

Feeling weak after hemodialysis treatments is a common experience of some hemodialysis patients. Many patients feel well after their treatments. They finish dialysis and rush off to work, leading a busy life. Other patients find that they must rest or lie down after their treatment but feel much stronger the day following their treatment. When we remove poisons and toxins during hemodialysis, we remove these substances from the blood. These poisons and toxins also are found in our brain. When we rapidly remove toxins from our bloodstream, there is a lag before they are removed from the brain. This lag is because the brain and the central nervous system are isolated from the circulation by a covering called the **meninges**. The meninges decrease the movement of substances in and out of the central nervous system. They form what doctors call the blood-brain barrier. When poisons and toxins are rapidly removed from the circulation during hemodialysis, the brain still contains a high concentration of poisons and toxins. Water will move through the blood-brain barrier faster than the poisons and toxins can move out. This causes swelling of the brain. This brain swelling occurs to a greater or lesser extent in every patient on hemodialysis.

Brain swelling during hemodialysis is known as the **disequilibrium syndrome**. Symptoms of the disequilibrium syndrome include headache, weakness, fatigue, nausea, and vomiting. In its extreme form, the patient can become unresponsive or even have a

Meninges

The three membranes that cover the brain and spinal cord. The meninges form a barrier between the central nervous system and the rest of the body, known as the blood-brain barrier.

Disequilibrium syndrome

A syndrome in which the rapid removal of poisons and toxins during hemodialysis results in less toxins being present in the blood than in the brain. This difference causes water to leave the blood stream and enter the central nervous system, leading to brain swelling. Symptoms include headache, nausea, vomiting, fatigue, and weakness. Most of these symptoms are gone by the next day. A severe disequilibrium syndrome can cause seizures and coma.

seizure. Fortunately, doctors know who is at risk for the disequilibrium syndrome, and the severe manifestations of the syndrome are rare. In its mild form, it can cause patients to feel washed out and weak. The swelling of the brain is usually gone by the next day, which is why patients feel better the day after their hemodialysis treatment. The disequilibrium syndrome does not occur in peritoneal dialysis because peritoneal dialysis is a gentle treatment and removes poisons and toxins more slowly over a longer time. This allows the brain to equilibrate slowly with the rest of the body, preventing brain swelling. Patients on nocturnal hemodialysis also do not suffer from the disequilibrium syndrome.

There are many other reasons why patients feel weak after dialysis. If you drink a large amount of liquid between treatments, the dialysis team may try to remove a large amount of fluid during hemodialysis, putting a tremendous strain on the heart and circulation and leading to low blood pressure or hypotension. This lowering of the blood pressure means there is less blood flowing to the brain, heart, and other vital organs of the body. Especially if you are older, or have heart disease or high blood pressure, this low blood pressure can make you feel weak and more debilitated. Some patients are better off removing less fluid, even if they are left with some swelling of the feet, which is called edema.

When you begin your hemodialysis treatment, your body has not adjusted to dialysis. Over time, most patients feel stronger after their dialysis treatment and adjust very well to hemodialysis. This adjustment period is not easy and can take up to 6 months' time. To feel stronger after your dialysis treatment, it is important to receive a good dialysis, which will keep the level of poisons and toxins lower in your body. When you have been having good hemodialysis treatments, there will be fewer poisons removed on each treatment, and this will decrease the amount of brain swelling that occurs. Achieving this means staying on dialysis longer and having a good access that will allow you to have a high flow of blood to the dialysis machine to remove more poisons and toxins. Feeling stronger on dialysis requires keeping to your renal diet and decreasing the amount of fluid you drink between treatments. This will lessen the chance of you developing a low blood pressure and feeling sick.

An exercise program is crucial to feeling stronger on dialysis.

An exercise program is crucial to feeling stronger on dialysis. Many patients begin an exercise program or physical therapy. They have an increased feeling of well-being, better endurance, and greater muscle strength that allows them to perform many of their most difficult daily tasks more easily. When they stop exercising, many patients feel weaker and more fatigued. An exercise program can make the difference between being an independent patient or one who is reliant on others. The psychological benefits of exercise are well known to athletes and doctors. Exercise stimulates endorphin release in the brain. Endorphins are chemical messengers released during pleasurable activities. In one study, patients who exercised have similar improvements in their depression as patients on antidepressants.

75. What will happen if there is an electrical power failure while I am on dialysis?

Electrical power is essential for hemodialysis treatments. Peritoneal dialysis is driven not by electricity but by gravity, so no electrical power is needed. In an emergency, peritoneal dialysis could be performed using flashlights for illumination without difficulty. Most hospitals have emergency generators because a loss of electrical power is extremely dangerous to patients on life support such as ventilators. Patients undergoing major surgery would also be in danger from power failure. Some hemodialysis units that are located in hospitals may be covered by their hospital emergency generator. Dialysis units in parts of the country that have frequent power outages due to storms and downed power lines may have emergency generators. Emergency generators do not cover most freestanding dialysis units.

All dialysis units have emergency plans to cope with electrical power failures. In the event of an electrical power failure, your dialysis machine would immediately stop and the blood flow out of your access would stop. All dialysis machines have a crank to manually turn the blood pump on the dialysis machine. This crank allows the dialysis staff to hand power the blood pump to return your blood to your body. Healthy patients may be able to help the staff in turning the crank to return their blood. Your dialysis unit will instruct you in the procedures to follow in case of emergency, which include what to do during electrical power failure, fire, and other emergencies.

My dialysis unit in Brooklyn experienced an electrical power failure on August 14, 2003, when the electrical grid powering the city and much of the northeastern United States went down. We had 18 patients on dialysis when the power went off, and all of them had their blood returned to their body using the blood pump crank. If it is not possible to return the blood in time, the

Electrical power failure is an inconvenience, not a true emergency.

blood loss will not be very significant and the chance of harm is low. The main adverse effect of electrical power failure is panic and fear in patients and staff. If you do have an electrical power failure in your unit, remain calm. If you are familiar with the emergency procedures to return your blood and disconnect from the dialysis machine, by all means follow them. If you are not comfortable with the emergency plan, wait patiently for the staff to return your blood and disconnect you from the hemodialysis machine. Electrical power failure is an inconvenience, not a true emergency.

76. Why do peritoneal dialysis patients develop peritonitis?

Peritonitis

An inflammation of the peritoneal membrane, which covers the intestines, caused by infection.

Peritonitis is one of the main complications of peritoneal dialysis. Peritonitis is an inflammation of the lining of the intestines. In most cases, peritonitis is caused by bacteria entering the abdomen through the peritoneal catheter. Some patients develop infections because of poor dialysis technique. Because the peritoneal catheter is tunneled through the skin and exits the abdomen, the most likely source of the bacteria is from the skin. To prevent infection, patients on peritoneal dialysis wear a mask while performing their dialysis. They carefully wash their hands with a bactericidal soap. Purell is a bactericidal solution that can be rubbed on the hands to decrease the chance of infection.

Peritoneal dialysis patients should shower and avoid bathtubs. Patients may swim in the ocean or in a private pool. They should avoid hot tubs, saunas, and jacuzzis because these warm environments promote the growth of bacteria on the skin. Patients perform exit site care every day. This involves swabbing the area where the catheter exits the skin with an antiseptic solution and applying a sterile dressing over the exit site. It is important that the catheter be securely taped to the abdomen to prevent it from twisting and turning with activity.

Symptoms of bacterial peritonitis are abdominal pain, fever, chills, and a cloudy peritoneal dialysate. It is important to recognize these signs of infection and to bring the dialysate to the peritoneal dialysis unit or to the emergency room if the unit is closed. The peritoneal dialysis fluid can be cultured by the laboratory to determine which bacteria are causing the infection. As part of the culture, the microbiology lab will test the bacteria causing the peritonitis to determine which antibiotics to use. A cell count will also be performed to measure the white blood cells in your dialysate. In 90% of peritonitis cases, the bacteria causing peritonitis are staphylococcus or streptococcus. These bacteria are normally present on our skin. The cell count and dialysate culture will guide peritoneal dialysis nurses' and physicians' choice of antibiotic. Most of the time the antibiotics will be given by injecting them into the dialysate, which is infused into the abdomen. The antibiotics will be rapidly delivered to the location where they are needed most. Many patients with bacterial peritonitis can be treated as an outpatient. If the peritonitis is severe, your doctor may want to admit you to the hospital.

Other causes of peritonitis in peritoneal dialysis patients are appendicitis, diverticulitis, and perforation of the bowel. The clue to these conditions is a dialysate culture with gram-negative organisms from the bowel, which are unusual in cases of peritonitis. Other clues are the failure of response to antibiotics. A CT scan of the abdomen can sometimes diagnose the problem and guide the treatment. Patients can have peritonitis due to fungi such as *Candida*. These patients have often had multiple courses of antibiotics. The peritoneal dialysis catheter should be removed in cases of fungal peritonitis. Antibiotics for fungal peritonitis can be given by mouth or intravenously.

As peritoneal dialysis has improved over the years, the frequency of peritonitis has decreased dramatically. Peritoneal dialysis programs are constantly working hard to decrease the rate of peritonitis in their patients. It is important to realize that hemodialysis patients can also have infections of their access with bacteria, which may result in their catheter or a-v graft being removed. A rare cause of peritonitis is an allergic reaction to dialysate. These patients have a high percentage of **eosinophils** in their cell count. Eosinophils are white blood cells that are frequently released during allergic reactions. Patients can also develop an infection around their peritoneal dialysis catheter, which is called a tunnel infection. Redness around the catheter exit site and drainage of pus or liquid around the catheter are signs of a tunnel infection. You will learn a great deal about peritonitis and catheter tunnel infections during your peritoneal dialysis training.

Eosinophils

White blood cells produced by bone marrow that are active in inflammation caused by allergic reactions as well as other diseases.

The large majority of patients with heart problems can be safely treated with hemodialysis and peritoneal dialysis.

77. Will my chest pain or angina get worse on dialysis?

Patients with heart problems are often concerned about the effect of dialysis on their cardiac condition. Beginning dialysis is stressful. The large majority of patients with heart problems can be safely treated with hemodialysis and peritoneal dialysis. It is important for your kidney doctor to be aware of your heart condition before you start dialysis and for you to talk to your cardiologist.

Your medications should be optimized so that you will have less of a chance of developing chest pain on dialysis. Many patients who develop chest pain or angina bring their nitroglycerine tablets with them while they are on hemodialysis. If they begin to experience chest pain, they can inform their nurse and immediately place a nitroglycerine tablet under their tongue. Oxygen is sometimes given to patients with heart problems while they receive their dialysis treatments to help prevent episodes of chest pain. Excessive weight gain and water intake between dialysis treatments are best avoided. Removing a great deal of fluid will put strain on your heart and precipitate an angina attack. It can also cause your heart to develop a rapid heart rate and low blood pressure. Patients with heart disease can develop atrial fibrillation or atrial flutter. These episodes of rapid heart rates often resolve by themselves when dialysis is stopped. Medication may be needed to control the heart rate.

Patients with chest pain, irregular heartbeats, or other cardiac symptoms should be carefully evaluated by a cardiologist or heart specialist. Many tests can be performed to determine if the blood vessels to the heart are blocked. If blockages exist, they can often be treated by inserting a balloon across the blockage and inflating it to open up the blocked artery. A cardiac stent or tube, is usually inserted to open the the blockage. This small tube will help prevent the blockage from returning at the same place. If the blockages are too numerous, heart bypass surgery can be done to improve blood flow to the heart. One of the advantages of heart surgery over cardiac stents is that the heart surgery patient does not need to take medications to prevent clotting of the stent. If a patient develops bleeding in the gastrointestinal tract or has had bleeding in the brain, it could be important to stop medications such as aspirin and Plavix, which interfere with platelet function.

Fortunately, medical science has made great strides in developing effective treatments for heart disease. These include medications that lower cholesterol, lower high blood pressure, improve heart failure, and treat angina. Medical devices such as pacemakers and implantable defibrillators can be used in dialysis patients to make sure the heart is beating properly. Revascularization procedures such as cardiac stents and bypass surgery can improve blood supply to the heart. Damaged heart valves can be repaired or replaced. All of these treatments can be successfully used in patients on dialysis. Treatments for heart disease are rapidly becoming more effective and safer, which will help dialysis patients live longer and have a better quality of life.

PART SEVEN

Dialysis: A Healthy Lifestyle

How can I lose weight as a dialysis patient?

Can dialysis patients participate in sports?

How will being a kidney dialysis patient affect my teeth?

More ...

78. Why do some patients do better on dialysis?

The effect of the psyche or the mind on physical illness should never be underestimated. Patients with a positive attitude do better.

This question of why there is variability in patient outcomes has intrigued doctors. When two patients who are the same age and have the same diagnosis, blood pressure, cholesterol level, financial resources, and support at home begin dialysis, why does one patient have a better outcome? Why do some patients survive longer on dialysis? This phenomenon has also been noticed in cancer patients, patients with infections such as pneumonia, and in patients with many chronic illnesses. The effect of the psyche or the mind on physical illness should never be underestimated. Patients with a positive attitude do better.

When it comes to dialysis, successful patients are those who are able to commit to the dialysis lifestyle. This is hard to do. Many patients with kidney failure have neglected their medical care in the past, leading to kidney damage. Patients may have not taken their medication regularly, kept their doctors' appointments, or stayed on their diet. Beginning dialysis treatments is a wake-up call for many patients. The message is, my health and life are important and I need to do a better job taking care of myself.

In some ways, committing to the dialysis lifestyle is like being a competitive athlete. There is a great deal of loss in beginning dialysis. Your time is not your own. You must show up for your treatments at the hemodialysis center or be on a schedule for your peritoneal dialysis exchanges. An athlete may not want to go to the pool for 2 hours of swimming laps followed by weight training, but he or she does it in pursuit of a goal. You cannot eat what you want as a dialysis patient. Athletes look at that big piece of chocolate cake for dessert and pass it by. They know if they gain weight they will run, bike, or swim slower. They are able to give up their immediate gratification for their long-term goals. They are committed to being the best they can be. Life on dialysis is full of choices. You can go to your treatment, or skip treatment or decrease your treatment time. You can stay on your diet, or eat what you want. You can remember to take your medication, or leave it in the pill container. Successful patients make their treatments time after time. They are not looking for ways to cut corners; they want to be the best they can be. This commitment is not easy or fun, but it will pay off in the long run. As a dialysis patient, you must ask yourself, "Will I do the minimum, or will I be the best I can be?"

Successful patients make their treatments time after time. They are not looking for ways to cut corners; they want to be the best they can be.

Patients on hemodialysis will do better if they have a good dialysis access. The most common complication in hemodialysis is access problems. Patients with catheters have a high rate of infection and scarring of the blood vessels. Arterial-venous grafts have a high rate of clotting or thrombosis and also are prone to infection. It is important to have an a-v fistula. This access is constructed of your own artery and vein, making it less likely to develop infection or clotting. The fistula takes a longer time to develop or mature. If you want to do well on hemodialysis, you should work with your vascular surgeon to develop an a-v fistula. A good a-v fistula with a good blood flow will help you clear more toxins and poisons from your bloodstream, and this will decrease the amount of complications you will have over many years. An a-v fistula will minimize interruptions in your dialysis treatments due to access failure. It will decrease the chance of an infection in your access spreading to other parts of your body. A good a-v fistula could last 20 years or more.

After access problems, the most common complications in dialysis patients relate to their cardiac health. Heart problems are more common in patients with kidney disease. This is because the risk factors for heart disease such as high blood pressure, diabetes, and elevated cholesterol levels are more common in patients with kidney disease. To do well long term on dialysis, you should do what you can to minimize these risks. If you are a smoker, you must try to stop smoking. Elevated blood pressure should be controlled with medication and diet. Diabetes should be treated aggressively. You will need specialized help from an **endocrinologist**. This doctor has special training in the evaluation and treatment of patients with diabetes and can work with your nephrologist to improve your blood sugars. Many new medications have recently become available to help you. The **diabetes nurse educator** is a nurse with special training in diabetes who can also work with you to help control your diabetes. Ask your nephrologist if a referral to these healthcare professionals would be appropriate for you. Medications to control cholesterol work well in dialysis patients. Your cholesterol should be measured at least once a year, and you should lower an elevated cholesterol with diet and medications. Dialysis patients with cardiovascular risk factors should be evaluated by a cardiologist. The cardiologist can help detect cardiac problems at an early stage by using noninvasive testing such as echocardiograms, stress tests, and nuclear scans. This early detection can help prevent cardiac problems before they happen and help keep you well.

Endocrinologist

A physician who has trained in internal medicine and who has received additional training in the treatment of patients with diabetes, thyroid disease, parathyroid disease, and other glandular disorders.

Diabetes nurse educator

A nurse who has obtained special training and certification in the evaluation and education of patients with diabetes.

79. How can I lose weight as a dialysis patient?

When we discuss weight with dialysis patients, there are several types of weight. One is the weight we lose on dialysis. This corresponds to the fluid removal. The other is what we call our **dry weight**. This corresponds to our weight after dialysis when we do not have extra fluid in our body. Dry weight is the target weight we are aiming for where we feel well and have good blood pressure control. The third weight is called **ideal body weight**. This weight is dependent on your age, height, and body build. Ideal body weights are different for men and women. This weight reflects a healthy weight for you. There are tables available for you to look up your ideal body weight. Your dietitian in the dialysis unit can tell you your ideal body weight. The ideal body weight is based on population studies. It can be used as a guide to determine if you are too light or too heavy. Most of us have a weight that we feel is appropriate for us. Our weight is influenced by cultural and familial factors. In some cultures, being heavy is considered a sign of good health and prosperity. A chubby baby with fat cheeks and fat arms and legs is thought to be healthy and doing well. If our parents are heavy, we are more likely to view a heavy body image as desirable or normal.

Being overweight may have several medical consequences, including elevated blood pressure and difficulty controlling diabetes. Being overweight can also put stress on our heart. It can cause our joints to wear out sooner because our knees and hips are carrying excess weight. Some patients who are very heavy may suffer from a syndrome called sleep apnea. These

Dry weight

The body weight of hemodialysis patients at the end of their hemodialysis treatment. The dry weight is determined by removing fluid until the blood pressure begins to fall.

Ideal body weight

Ideal body weight is dependent upon your age, height, body, build, and sex, and is based on the measured average weight of normal individuals. Ideal body weights can be found in published tables, which are available from your kidney dietitian.

patients have difficulty breathing when they fall asleep. The tube that carries air to the lungs (the trachea) can be blocked, causing the patient to wake up many times during the night and preventing restful sleep. For all these reasons, kidney dialysis patients who are over-weight are often encouraged by their physicians to lose weight.

Losing weight as a dialysis patient is similar to losing weight in people not on dialysis. It requires commit-ment. Decreasing the calories you eat every day and increasing your activity level with exercise is the stan-dard approach. The dietitian at the dialysis unit can help you choose foods that have high nutritional value and fewer calories. Many different diets are advertised in the media for losing weight. Many of these diets are very restrictive. People frequently lose a lot of weight in a short time only to gain it back. Diets that aim for a slower loss of weight by changing your eating habits are more likely to be effective long term. It is impor-tant to check with your nephrologist and dietitian before starting any diet to see if the diet is safe for kid-ney dialysis patients. Diet pills are generally not a good idea for dialysis patients, as they can have some serious side effects. In extreme cases of obesity, weight loss surgery called bariatric surgery can be performed to band the stomach, causing a decrease in your ability to eat too much. Intestinal bypass operations may also be used to treat obesity. These procedures are used as a last resort when dieting and medical management has failed.

Most people find it difficult to lose weight alone. Sup-port groups such as Weight Watchers have been suc-cessful in helping people lose weight because they have a structure and a great deal of positive support. It is easier to keep your diet when you have friends who are also trying to lose weight. If your spouse, significant other, or other family members are also overweight, consider encouraging them to join you in your weight loss program. This may make it easier to change your eating habits and to limit some of the high-calorie food that comes into your home. If you do buy high-calorie foods as a treat, consider buying a smaller container. Avoid extra large sizes of cookies, chips, candy, and cakes, even if they cost the same as the small package. This way if you go off your diet, you will not eat as much of these foods. Exercising is also easier to do with others. If you have a regular appointment with a friend to walk, jog, bike ride, or go to the gym, you are more likely to exercise. The best results in losing weight are because of changes in a person's lifestyle that result in a gradual loss of weight.

80. Can dialysis patients participate in sports?

Dialysis patients can participate in a wide range of sports and activities. Studies have shown that regular exercise and physical activity increase patients' sense of well-being, decrease fatigue, improve depression, lower blood pressure, and improve blood sugar control in diabetic patients. It is also fun, especially if you exercise with someone else. It is important to discuss your sports plans with your doctor before you start your exercise program.

Hemodialysis patients with catheters cannot get their catheters wet because of the risks of infection. These patients should not participate in swimming and water sports. Hemodialysis patients with fistulas and grafts can swim and get their access wet. Peritoneal dialysis patients can swim in the ocean or a private pool. Public pools may have a higher bacteria count in the water and are not advised. After swimming, patients on peritoneal dialysis should perform their exit site care. The peritoneal dialysis catheter should be securely taped to the abdomen during swimming or exercise to prevent irritation of the access site.

Patients on peritoneal dialysis should exercise with their abdomen drained of peritoneal dialysis fluid. They should not perform abdominal exercises such as crunches, sit-ups, or leg lifts. They should perform exit site care after their workout because sweat will help bacteria grow on the skin.

Exercises that increase cardiac function such as walking, biking, tennis, and jogging are preferred to exercises that require lifting weights.

Hemodialysis patients with fistulas and grafts are discouraged from lifting weights greater than 20 pounds with their access arm. Lifting heavy weights in general is not the best exercise for dialysis patients because lifting has been associated with increasing blood pressure during the lift. Exercises that increase cardiac function such as walking, biking, tennis, and jogging are preferred to exercises that require lifting weights. Calisthenics are good exercises for dialysis patients. After beginning dialysis, many patients feel fatigued and weak. You should decrease the intensity and level of your activity. If you are used to walking a mile a day, you may want to walk for a quarter of a mile for one week and see how you feel. If you feel capable of more activity, double the distance every week. If you are used to playing tennis for an hour, try 10 or 20 minutes at first. Increase your activity level as long as you are feeling well. It is not important how much exercise you can do, the important point is to start. As we get older, we become more sedentary. We lose the simple joy of shooting a basketball, catching a fly ball, or ice-skating. We all have a thousand reasons to avoid being active. Inertia is the most powerful force in the universe.

It takes effort to overcome the negative feelings of "I cannot do this anymore," "I'm too old," "People will laugh at me," and so forth. Try to overcome these negative feelings. Be prepared for failure. If you become dizzy or feel faint, stop, lie down, and rest. Regroup. Ask your doctor about your symptoms. He or she may recommend changes in your exercise regimen that will help you be active without these symptoms. Avoid exercising in very high temperatures that can lead to dehydration and heat stroke. Use common sense in your exercise. If you bike, rollerblade, or ski, wear a helmet. This is good advice for everyone, on dialysis or not. Do not swim alone. Use the buddy system. Try a new sport. Use beginning dialysis as an excuse to treat yourself to something you always wanted to try but never had the time to try. You need to be active to do well on dialysis. Take lessons to make sure you are using your sports equipment safely and are getting the most out of your exercise time. Have fun!

Erick Lucero writes:

I have always been an active person. At age 12, I became interested in calisthenics at school because I wanted to play baseball. I did exercises that got my legs strong because this would improve the power of my hitting and fielding. I played on traveling baseball teams since I was 12. Later on, I played in baseball leagues on weekends. I play second base. On June 4, 2007, I played for my team. On June 6, I started hemodialysis. At first, I was very weak. Little by little, I began throwing the ball around. In October, I was

*able to play the last two league games of the season. My
team needed me, and they gladly welcomed me back.*

*The best exercise for dialysis patients is walking. You can
do this even if you are not feeling your best. Walking in the
park is my favorite. Walking strengthens your leg muscles.
If your legs are good, everything else will follow. Stretching
is very important for hemodialysis patients. On hemodialysis, you are sitting still for 4 hours. Stretching will make
your muscles feel better and decrease cramps on dialysis.*

81. How can I keep my bones strong?

Keeping your bones strong requires good nutrition and
regular exercise. In addition, kidney dialysis patients
are especially susceptible to a type of weakening of the
bones that is due to kidney disease. This weakening of
the bones is known as **metabolic bone disease** or renal
osteodystrophy. Bone problems begin early on in kidney failure, before patients begin dialysis treatments.
Most of the calcium and phosphorus in our bodies
reside in our bones. Our bones are a large reservoir of
these important minerals. As kidney function declines,
phosphorus levels rise in the blood. The elevated phosphorus combines with the calcium in the blood and
pushes the calcium back into the bones. As a result,
the level of calcium in the blood decreases.

Metabolic bone disease

Bone disease in renal patients is caused by reabsorption of bone by cells called osteo-clasts whose growth is stimulated by PTH. Patients with bone disease can have bone pain and are more prone to frac-tures. Also called renal osteodystrophy.

Another reason for low calcium is decreased vitamin D
activity in kidney patients. The kidney is necessary for
the production of active vitamin D. Vitamin D helps
absorb calcium that is in the food we eat from the gastrointestinal tract. When the calcium level falls, cells in
the parathyroid glands, called chief cells, sense the low
calcium level in the blood. The parathyroid glands are
four small glands that are located on the thyroid gland

in front of the neck, at the windpipe near the bulge called the Adam's apple. When the calcium level is low, the chief cells signal the parathyroid glands to produce more PTH. PTH travels through the body in the blood, signaling the gastrointestinal tract to absorb more calcium and telling the kidneys to stop eliminating calcium from the body. PTH also tells cells in the bones called osteoclasts to start releasing calcium from the bones. If the calcium remains low for a long time, the parathyroid gland grows larger and produces abnormally high levels of PTH. The high PTH level can cause too much calcium to leave our bones, resulting in bones that have less structural material holding us up. If the bones lose calcium, they are more susceptible to fractures. Patients develop changes of the bones of their fingers and collarbones that can be seen on x-rays. The most important evidence that bone problems are occurring is from blood tests. Calcium and phosphorus levels are measured every month in dialysis patients to evaluate bone health. Another blood test, alkaline phosphatase can be elevated if the bone is being reabsorbed too rapidly. PTH is also measured on a regular basis.

The first step in maintaining good bone health is to keep your phosphorus level low. This can be done by decreasing intake of phosphorus-containing foods like milk products and beans. Your dietitian will be reviewing these foods with you on a regular basis. Medications can also be helpful in decreasing the absorption of phosphorus from the gastrointestinal tract. Phosphate binders such as PhosLo, which contain calcium acetate, and calcium carbonate binders such as Tums contain calcium that binds phosphorus. Renagel contains sevelamer hydrochloride as a binder. Another binder is Fosrenol, which contains lanthanum carbonate. Fosrenol is a chewable tablet. All the phosphorus binders are taken by mouth and trap phosphorus in the gastrointestinal tract. It is important to remember to decrease the phosphorus in the diet. Vitamin D analogs are also frequently used to keep patients' bones strong. They work by increasing the absorption of calcium from the gastrointestinal tract. They also suppress the production and secretion of PTH. Vitamin D is available as capsules taken by mouth and also as an injection that can be given during the hemodialysis treatment. Some Vitamin D analogs are Rocaltrol, Hectorol, Zemplar, and Calcijex.

Sensipar (cinacalcet hydrochloride) is a medication used to treat kidney dialysis patients who are at risk for developing metabolic bone disease. It is different from other medications that treat bone disease because it is the only medication of its kind available. Sensipar decreases PTH as well as calcium and phosphorus. Vitamin D analogs can decrease PTH, but they can also cause a rise in serum calcium. PTH is produced by the parathyroid glands that are located in the neck. Most people have four parathyroid glands that sit on the thyroid gland. The parathyroid glands have chief cells that have calcium-sensing receptors on their surface. Sensipar increases the sensitivity of these receptors to the calcium in the blood. Sensipar causes a decrease in the PTH secretion as well as a decrease in calcium and phosphorus. This is beneficial because decreasing the amount of calcium circulating in the blood can decrease the calcium that ends up being deposited in blood vessels and other organs of the body.

When Sensipar first became available, it was used in the most difficult cases in patients who had very high

PTH levels. Some of these patients were having multiple fractures and were facing surgical removal of the parathyroid glands. This operation is called a parathyroidectomy. Sensipar was effective in reducing the PTH level in many of these patients and some of them were able to avoid parathyroid surgery. As doctors used Sensipar and found that it was well tolerated by most patients, it began to be used in more patients.

The most frequent side effects of Sensipar are an upset stomach, nausea, vomiting, diarrhea, and muscle cramps. Sensipar comes as a tablet and is available in 30-mg, 60-mg, and 90-mg strengths. Most patients start with the 30-mg tablet. Sensipar is absorbed in 2 to 6 hours and should be taken with food. It is important before you begin taking Sensipar to tell your doctor if you have a history of seizures or liver disease, if you are on any psychiatric medications, or if you are pregnant or are planning to become pregnant. Blood tests including calcium, phosphorus, and PTH levels are followed carefully when you take Sensipar to see if your calcium level falls. Sensipar can be safely used with phosphate binders, as well as vitamin D analogs. Most patients on dialysis are on several medications to prevent bone problems.

When I first started my career treating kidney dialysis patients over 25 years ago, bone disease was a major problem for patients. Many patients had multiple fractures, bone pain, and spontaneous rupture of tendons. Surgery to remove the parathyroid glands was the only option to treat their severe bone disease. Fortunately, we have safe and effective medications that have resulted in better and safer treatment for metabolic bone disease and an improved quality of life for our patients on dialysis.

Do not be discouraged if phosphorus and calcium balance is very confusing to you. It is common for nursing and medical students to have difficulty understanding these concepts. The scientific names are also often overwhelming to patients. Try to concentrate on measures that will keep your phosphorus level normal. You will be reviewing this important subject many times in the future with your nurse, doctor, and dietitian.

82. Why is taking care of my eyes important as a dialysis patient?

We often take for granted our most precious sense, our eyesight. Patients on dialysis have an increased risk of vision loss. This is, in part, due to the fact that about 45% of patients on dialysis have diabetes. Diabetes affects the blood vessels in the kidneys and the eyes at the same time. The first sign of diabetes affecting the eyes is the enlargement of the veins at the back of the eye called the retina. These and other changes in the blood vessels can be seen during an examination by an ophthalmologist or an optometrist. These changes are called retinopathy. As the circulation to the back of the eye gets worse, new blood vessels grow in the retina. Blood vessels can bleed into the back of the eye causing an acute loss of vision. Over time, the blood in the back of the eye can cause scarring and further damage to the retina resulting in permanent loss of vision. Fortunately, damage to the eyes from diabetes can be prevented by careful control of the blood sugar. Damage to the retina can be treated by ophthalmologists with laser treatments. Laser treatments involve exposing damaged areas of the retina to laser light that is able to decrease the growth of new blood vessels. Laser treatments are done in the office and do not require the patient to be admitted to the hospital overnight.

Glaucoma is a group of eye diseases affecting the optic nerve, which is a bundle of nerves that enters the back of the eye and carries visual information from the eyes to our brain. Glaucoma is usually associated with an increased pressure in the eye. More than 2 million Americans over the age of 40 have some form of glaucoma. Risk factors for glaucoma include a family history of glaucoma, black or Hispanic ancestry, diabetes, and hypertension. Glaucoma is diagnosed during a visit to your ophthalmologist or optometrist. These eye doctors will measure the pressure in your eye, examine the optic nerve, and may measure the thickness of your cornea, which is the clear front surface of your eyes. Treatment for glaucoma is usually eye drops to decrease the pressure in the eye. Some forms of severe glaucoma are treated with eye surgery.

Age-related macular degeneration is a common cause of visual loss due to damage to the macula, which is the center of the retina. A healthy macula is needed for clear vision for activities such as reading, driving, recognizing faces, and observing fine details of objects. Macular degeneration generally begins after age 50. More than 14% of patients over the age of 70 suffer from some degree of macular degeneration. Other risk factors besides age include smoking, a family history of macular degeneration, and prolonged sun exposure. It is important not to smoke, and to wear hats and sunglasses to decrease sun exposure to your eyes, and to eat foods such as fresh fruits and vegetables rich in carotenoids, lutens, vitamin C, and vitamin E to decrease your chance of developing macular degeneration as you age. Foods rich in omega-3 fatty acids are also thought to decrease macular degeneration. Your renal dietitian can help you select foods that are part of the renal diet and good for your eyesight.

Dialysis patients should have an eye examination at least once a year. Many patients with diabetes, glaucoma, and macular degeneration should be followed more frequently. Another good practice is to wear glasses and sunglasses that have UV light protection to prevent the formation of cataracts. It is important to wear eye protection when working with tools or participating in sports. Eye guards are protective glasses made of a plastic called polycarbonate. Sports which have a high rate of eye injury include basketball, baseball, water sports, and racquet sports such as tennis, racquetball, and squash. Chemical burns of the eyes from household products such as drain and floor cleaners are common accidents and care should be used when handling these products. Protecting your vision as a kidney patient will help you maintain a good quality of life and decrease your dependency on others.

83. Why is it important to take my medications as a dialysis patient?

Many patients who begin dialysis treatments wonder why they still have to take medication. The average dialysis patient takes between 8 and 12 different pills a day. Taking this amount of medication is difficult for many patients. Dialysis is an imperfect treatment. The normal kidney performs hundreds of different tasks every day. These tasks involve cleaning the blood, metabolizing medications, stimulating the bone marrow to produce red blood cells, activating vitamin D, and regulating blood pressure. The hemodialysis machine and peritoneal dialysis only clean the blood. They can remove some medications. Other functions of the kidney are replaced by medications. To regulate your blood pressure, you will need to take blood pressure medications. To lower your phosphorus level, you will need to take phosphate binders. You will receive erythropoietin injections if you have a low blood count as well as injections of vitamin D. If you are a diabetic, you will continue to take your diabetes pills and injections of insulin. Many patients with diabetes need less medication because the kidneys metabolize the insulin your body produces. As your kidneys become diseased, there is more insulin available to decrease your blood sugar level. Some patients with type II diabetes can come off their diabetes medications. Patients may take medication for their heart to prevent heart attacks, such as aspirin, Plavix, beta blockers, ACE inhibitors, and nitrates. An elevated blood cholesterol is associated with kidney failure and needs to be treated with medication when diet alone is not successful. Bowel complaints such as heartburn and constipation are common in kidney patients. It is easy to see how the number of medications adds up quickly.

It is important to take your medications as a kidney dialysis patient because you will decrease the chances of having a complication that will decrease the quality or length of your life. When you are faced with taking an additional medication, it is important that you learn the reason for the medication from your doctor. The more knowledge you have, the better job you will do taking those pills. Dialysis patients often have several doctors and can end up taking two medications for the same problem. Ask your nephrologist if you can take medicines that can be taken once a day rather than two or three times a day. Many medications have a time-release form that allows you to take them once

It is important to take your medications as a kidney dialysis patient because you will decrease the chances of having a complication that will decrease the quality or length of your life.

a day. It may be possible to simplify by taking higher doses of one or two blood pressure medications and eliminating the third antihypertensive. Some medications are available in an adhesive patch that is applied to the skin. An example is the antihypertensive clonidine, which is available in a patch called Catapress TTS. The Catapress TTS patch is applied once a week. If you are taking clonidine twice a day, that is 14 less pills a week to swallow. Patches are especially useful for confused patients who may not remember to take their medication regularly and patients who do not like taking their pills.

If you are very overweight, the best way to reduce your medications is to lose weight. Many medical problems such as diabetes, hypertension, and elevated cholesterol get better with changes in diet. Increasing the time you spend on dialysis may help normalize your blood pressure and phosphorus level. Patients on daily dialysis therapies such as peritoneal dialysis, nocturnal dialysis, and daily home dialysis often are able to stop some of their blood pressure medication and phosphate binders. Perhaps one of these therapies is best for you.

84. My cholesterol is elevated. Is this a concern?

Cholesterol is a hot topic for everyone. An elevated cholesterol level is associated with hardening of the arteries called atherosclerosis. This hardening of the arteries causes blockages in the arteries to major important organs such as the heart, brain, bowels, arms, legs, and kidneys. If you develop a blockage to the heart, which is called angina, you may have chest pain. If the blockage is very severe, it may lead to a heart attack, which causes a portion of the heart muscle to die. This heart muscle injury is not reversible. If the blockage occurs to the brain, a stroke may occur. Blockages to the legs can cause pain in the calves while walking. Physicians have developed ingenious ways of bypassing these blockages with surgery and other techniques. Coronary bypass surgery for blockages of arteries to the heart involves taking veins in the legs and bypassing the blockage by creating a new tube to carry blood to the heart. Other procedures have been developed to improve circulation to the brain, legs, and kidneys. These procedures are truly wonderful and in some cases lifesaving. It would be better to prevent the blockages caused by hardening of the arteries due to atherosclerosis, which is why everyone is so concerned about cholesterol. An elevated cholesterol level is a major risk factor for developing hardening of the arteries that causes blockages. Other risk factors are high blood pressure, smoking, diabetes, and a family history of hardening of the arteries.

Kidney patients are prone to high cholesterol levels due to several causes. The most common cause of kidney failure is diabetes. Diabetic patients are more likely to have high cholesterol, especially if their diabetes is poorly controlled. Many kidney diseases cause high cholesterol. Patients in the pre-dialysis period with a large amount of protein loss in their urine have high cholesterol because the liver is making more cholesterol along with the protein albumin. Every patient with kidney problems should have their cholesterol measured. The total cholesterol level was the first screening test available. It is best to measure your cholesterol before you have eaten. The fasting cholesterol level will be an accurate measure of your cholesterol. Cholesterol levels rise after your eat. If you have risk factors for hardening of the arteries, it is generally recommended that your fasting total cholesterol be less than 200.

When we measure cholesterol, we typically order a panel of tests, often called the **lipid profile**. The lipid profile contains the total cholesterol level and the triglyceride level, which measures another fat in the blood. An important component of the total cholesterol level is the **low-density lipoprotein** level, referred to as **LDL**. The LDL level is associated with the bad blockages that cause so many problems. In patients with hardening of their arteries, it is recommended that your LDL level be below 100. The **high-density lipoprotein** level, **HDL**, is known as the good cholesterol. A low level of HDL is associated with hardening of the arteries and blockages. A high level of HDL protects people from developing hardening of the arteries. Exercise will raise HDL levels. If your total cholesterol level is high because your HDL is also high, you may not need treatment for a high cholesterol level.

Treatment for high cholesterol begins with diet. Meat, especially organ meat like liver, is high in cholesterol. Some fish, like swordfish, have a lot of cholesterol. Milk, ice cream, and cheese have a large amount of cholesterol. Your kidney dietitian will guide you on your low-cholesterol diet. If diet fails, there are medications available to decrease cholesterol. The statins are a class of medication that work by inhibiting HMG-CoA reductase, which helps synthesize cholesterol in the liver. Some statins are Zocor (simvastatin), Lipitor (atorvastatin), Pravacol (pravastatin), Crestor (rosuvastatin), Welchol (colesevelam), and Lescol (fluvastatin). Another medication for high cholesterol is niacin.

Lipid profile

A lipid profile is a series of blood tests that include total cholesterol, HDL cholesterol, LDL cholesterol, and triglycerides. It is used to evaluate patients for their risk of developing atherosclerosis.

Low-density lipoprotein (LDL)

Composed of proteins, triglycerides, and cholesterol bound together in the blood. A high LDL level is associated with atherosclerosis.

High-density lipoprotein (HDL)

The "good cholesterol" in our blood that protects us from heart disease and other vascular problems. A high level of HDL is protective, and it can be increased by exercising, eating foods such as garlic and onions, and by taking certain medications.

Many people are resistant to taking medications for an elevated cholesterol level. They are not convinced that treatment will be beneficial and will decrease the chances of a serious heart problem or stoke. The benefits of treatment for a high cholesterol level have been shown in many studies with different populations of patients in varying countries. Treatment is not without risk. Statins have risks of liver problems as well as muscle cramps and more serious muscle damage called rhabdomyolysis. It is important to have a frank discussion with your doctor to decide the best course of action for you if you have an elevated cholesterol level. Most people tolerate medications for elevated cholesterol without side effects.

85. How can I live longer as a dialysis patient?

The strategy to live longer as a dialysis patient is to modify the risk factors for the most common causes of demise in dialysis patients, which are cardiac disease and stroke. This means maintaining ideal body weight, controlling blood pressure and cholesterol, treating diabetes, not smoking, and having a regular evaluation with your doctor regarding these risk factors. You do not have to be perfect. You should strive to make improvements in these areas. For example, many people feel they are so heavy that it is no use losing weight. The reality is that losing as little as 5 pounds has beneficial effects on lowering blood pressure. It is important to set realistic goals and reward yourself when you achieve them. If your goal is to lose 40 pounds, there is less of a chance to meet this goal than 5 pounds. After you lose the first 5 pounds, try to lose the next 5 pounds.

Exercise is an important habit to develop. I was on a vacation in France several years ago and was waiting outside in my rented car for my wife to come out of a store. I watched an elderly woman come out of a butcher shop with her purchases. She placed her package in the basket of her bicycle and rode away. I immediately understood why life expectancy is longer in some countries. That woman has probably been riding her bicycle for 75 years. In most instances, we can fit exercise into our daily routine. Park your car 5 blocks from your house and try to go for a walk every day. Use the stairs instead of the elevator. Realize that exercise is best approached in small bits. Exercising for five or ten minutes is better than no exercise at all.

Dialysis patients can live longer by paying attention to their access. If they have a good access, such as an a-v fistula, they can receive better dialysis. Good dialysis is associated with living longer and with less complications of renal failure such as neuropathy. An a-v fistula is less likely to become infected than a hemodialysis catheter. If you are on peritoneal dialysis, ask your doctor how you can increase the amount of dialysis you receive. This may involve increasing the amount of dialysate in your peritoneal dialysis exchange. Avoid missing dialysis or not completing a peritoneal dialysis exchange. If you skip one peritioneal dialysis exchange, you are only receiving 75% of your dialysis for the day. If you miss one hemodialysis treatment, you are missing one-third of your dialysis for that week. Ask your doctor if you are getting enough dialysis. Should you increase your time on dialysis or be treated with a hemodialysis dialyzer with a larger clearance? These questions are best discussed in your doctor's office or during your care plan meeting with the dialysis team.

Patients on dialysis need to be flexible to live longer. You may be faced with changes in your medical condition, develop complications, or need emergency procedures to fix your access. The ability to accept these changes and develop a therapeutic alliance with the dialysis team will improve your chance of long-term survival as a dialysis patient. You may arrive at the dialysis unit before a vacation or other important event and be told that your catheter is infected and must be removed. The ability to understand your dialysis treatment and to respond to crisis will decrease your chances of having a complication that could be life threatening. Try to understand what your doctor and the dialysis team are saying about your problems. Evaluate the information, and adjust your behavior to overcome the obstacle in your way. Be flexible. Stay focused on the big picture.

Patients on dialysis need to be flexible to live longer.

86. How can I avoid being depressed as a dialysis patient?

Being depressed is a normal part of starting dialysis. Being dependent on dialysis treatments to live is very scary. Most patients feel their life is over when they begin dialysis. As they adjust to their treatment and feel better physically, they become more hopeful and realize their life is not over but is continuing in a new way. The ability to accept the dialysis lifestyle and go on with your life by making plans for the future is an important milestone in adjusting to dialysis.

Some of the depression dialysis patients face is due to the poisons and toxins present in kidney failure. If we perform an **electroencephalogram (EEG)** on dialysis

Electroencephalogram (EEG)

A medical test in which electrical impulses generated by the brain are recorded by attaching electrodes to the scalp.

patients, we find slowing of their electrical impulses. This typical change in the EEG of dialysis patients is due to the poisons and toxins of kidney failure. These changes are reversed by a successful kidney transplant. Several patients who I observed in the pre-dialysis phase of their kidney failure became depressed when they began hemodialysis. When they received a kidney transplant, they reverted to their previous cheerful, positive personality. It is important to realize that the depression is not your fault.

It is important to realize that the depression is not your fault.

The first thing to do if you find yourself depressed as a dialysis patient is to review your medications with your doctor. Many medications such as sleeping pills, pain medications, some antihypertensives, and medications for ulcers or heartburn can affect your mental function. Medications tend to accumulate in dialysis patients because they metabolize and eliminate medications from the body more slowly than patients not on dialysis. We do not think of alcohol as a medication, but it can increase depression. If you are drinking alcohol, discuss this with your doctor to see if it is increasing your depression.

Exercise can help decrease depression in dialysis patients. Athletes talk about the runner's high. This feeling is due to substances called endorphins, which are released by the brain during intense exercise. These substances cause a sense of well-being and encourage continued exercise. Exercise improves self-esteem, gets you out of the house, and gives you something to do if you have taken time off to adjust to dialysis. Never underestimate the benefits of exercise in your life.

If you continue to be depressed for 6 months after beginning dialysis, or if your feelings of depression are very severe, discuss the possible need for medication and psychiatric consultation with your doctor. Many patients on dialysis benefit a great deal from antidepressants. These medications are taken by mouth and work well in patients on dialysis. Most patients on dialysis who are treated with antidepressants are able to stop them after their depression improves. These medications are safe, effective, and can make life more rewarding if your depression is severe.

Patients with a history of depression before they developed kidney failure can be safely and successfully treated with dialysis. It is important to make sure your psychologist or psychiatrist talks to your nephrologist and maintains communication during your adjustment to dialysis. Some medications for depression such as lithium need to be adjusted or stopped when you develop kidney failure.

Discuss your feelings with your family, significant other, and the dialysis team. Many patients with depression improve because they share their feelings with dialysis patients they encounter in the waiting room of the dialysis unit. The knowledge that you are not alone in being depressed as a dialysis patient and that this is a common response to illness and dialysis treatments can be helpful in decreasing feelings of depression.

When you start dialysis, talk to other patients who are on dialysis. They have faced the same problems you face and have a helpful perspective. Often their stories will give you insight into your own adjustment to dialysis. Most patients starting dialysis feel alone. They speak to their nephrologist, nurse, family, but nothing has the same impact as talking to a fellow dialysis patient. They will help you overcome your depression. Make sure to listen to patients around you in the dialysis center waiting room. Their insight, advice, and support is invaluable.

87. What medications should I avoid as a dialysis patient?

Dialysis patients take a great deal of medication to help replace the function of their kidneys. Often busy physicians feel obligated to prescribe another medication for each new complaint. Many complaints may be due to a side effect of a medication that is then treated with another medication. An example of this is giving a patient painkillers such as codeine or oxycodone for the relief of chronic pain such as arthritis, back pain, or headache. These medications, called opiates, frequently cause side effects such as nausea, vomiting, and constipation. The best thing to do if these symptoms occur is to stop the medication. Stool softeners for constipation and Pepcid or Nexium for nausea and vomiting are frequently prescribed, but they do not get to the root of the problem, which is a drug side effect. It is a good practice to limit pain medication containing opiates to the least amount that can control pain. Many medications are metabolized and eliminated from the body more slowly in kidney dialysis patients, resulting in higher levels of medication in the blood of kidney patients than in people who have normal renal function. This high level of medication can make side effects more likely. With constant use, patients develop **tolerance** to the medication. This means that more medication is needed to get the same reduction in pain. Other approaches to chronic pain such as medications

Tolerance

The need for an increasing amount of medication to produce the same effect over time. A common example is the need to use more pain medication to relieve chronic pain.

that are not opiates, physical therapy, heat, and massage can often be just as effective with fewer side effects. Sleeping pills can also accumulate in the blood of dialysis patients. The side effects of sleeping pills include an inability to wake up in times of danger, such as during a fire in your house. Sleeping pills can cause depression, anxiety, difficulty concentrating, and other problems. They are best used for a short time, if at all.

Medications for diabetes have to be carefully monitored in dialysis patients. Some medications such as Glucophage should not be used at all. The kidney metabolizes insulin, and patients with kidney failure often need less insulin when their kidney disease progresses to prevent the blood sugar from falling too low. Medications called sulfonylureas used to treat type II diabetes are removed from the body by the kidneys. These drugs can accumulate in patients with kidney failure and cause low blood sugar for several days until they are eliminated from the body.

Lithium, a drug used to treat manic depression, is excreted by the kidney and should not be used in patients on dialysis. Most other medications for psychiatric conditions can be safely used in dialysis patients.

Get in the habit of asking your doctor the reason for any new medications that are prescribed. Ask your doctor if the medication is important or if you can do without it. Most dialysis patients end up taking 8 to 12 different medications a day. Many patients are overwhelmed by the number of medications and forget or are unable to take all of them on a regular basis. By trying to take medications that are important in maintaining good health and avoiding unnecessary medications, you will decrease the chances of side effects and drug interactions. You will also be more successful in taking your medications at the right time and be less likely to skip a dose.

88. How will being a kidney dialysis patient affect my teeth?

Patients with kidney problems have more dental problems than patients not on dialysis. This may be because of an increase in the urea and phosphate in the secretions of the salivary glands in the mouth. Patients on dialysis have more plaque and **calculus** formation from bacteria on their teeth. Plaque is a layer of saliva, bacteria, protein, and sugar that forms a film that covers the teeth. When calcium is deposited in the center of the plaque, calculus is formed. Calculus is from the Latin word meaning pebble or stone. Calculus is more difficult to remove. Plaque and calculus can cause an inflammation of the gums, which is called gingivitis. If not treated, gingivitis can lead to serious dental infections and tooth loss. Kidney dialysis patients also have decreased salivary gland secretion, which can lead to parotid gland infection. They can have demineralization of the jawbone due to renal bone disease. Bone demineralization can lead to periodontal disease (disease of the gums), which can cause loose teeth. Dialysis patients are more susceptible to infections of the mouth from *Candida*. They also can get ulcers of the mouth.

The most effective way of removing plaque and calculus from the teeth is brushing and flossing your teeth

Calculus

Comes from the Latin word for stone. A kidney stone is sometimes referred to as a calculus. The term is also used by dentists to describe a calcified layer of saliva, bacteria, protein, and sugar covering the teeth.

at least twice a day. However, brushing alone cannot remove all of the plaque formed daily on your teeth. Plaque is also removed when your teeth are cleaned at your regular visit to your dentist. One study by dentists involving kidney dialysis patients showed that one-half of the patients never brushed their teeth or had regular visits to a dentist. When dialysis patients go to the dentist, it is more likely to be for a specific complaint or problem, not for prevention. This may be because dialysis patients are busy with other health concerns. They may not regard good dental care as a priority. While dental care is also expensive, it is much easier and cheaper to prevent dental disease than to treat it. It is important to keep your teeth and mouth as healthy as possible. Ask your dentist or hygienist to demonstrate proper brushing and flossing techniques. Poor dentition and periodontal or gum disease can interfere with your nutrition, require you to have extensive painful dental procedures, or cause infection in your mouth to spread to other areas of your body such as your lungs and heart. Patients who eat large amounts of sweets and carbohydrates are more likely to have tooth decay. When we eat food with high sugar content, bacteria in the mouth ferment the sugar, which produces acid. The acid encourages the formation of dental caries, also known as cavities. Good oral hygiene will help you live a longer and healthier life on dialysis.

Good oral hygiene will help you live a longer and healthier life on dialysis.

Dialysis patients can safely undergo most dental procedures. Make sure your nephrologist knows when you are scheduled for your dental procedure. It is important to tell your dentist if you are taking any blood thinners like Coumadin, aspirin, Plavix, Persantine, or

Aggrenox, which could cause more bleeding. Also, mention allergies or drug reactions to antibiotics or pain medication. Remind your dentist that the best day for dental procedures is the day after your dialysis treatment. Many dialysis patients receive prophylactic antibiotics during their dental work, which may decrease the chance of an infection in the dialysis access or other areas of the body caused by bacteria entering the bloodstream during the procedure. Dialysis patients are at a somewhat higher risk of complications from general anesthesia. If you need general anesthesia for your dental work, you might want to have it as an outpatient in a hospital setting. If you develop a complication, your nephrologist and other doctors may be more available than in the dentist's office.

Erick Lucero writes:

I began going to the dentist before I was on dialysis. My sister-in-law is a dental hygienist, and she got me to go to the dentist. Before I was on dialysis, I was taking a medication called cyclosporine to help prevent my kidneys from getting worse. The cyclosporine made my gums swell. My dentist explained the need for kidney patients to have regular dental checkups. This got me in the routine of going to the dentist every 6 months. I used to brush my teeth once a day. Now I brush my teeth three times a day (after every meal) and floss. I have a toothbrush I keep at work. Many dialysis patients avoid going to the dentist because they are worried about receiving more bad news about their health. Good oral hygiene is a good thing. It helps you feel better about your health.

89. Why do I have problems sleeping at night?

Most dialysis patients have difficulty sleeping at night at one time or another. The sleep-wake cycle, called the circadian rhythm, that regulates our sleep cycle is disturbed in dialysis patients because of the toxins and poisons in their bodies that are not removed by dialysis. Dialysis patients tend to nap and feel tired in the day and are wide awake at night. They have difficulty falling asleep. It is important to avoid napping during the day, which will make the problem worse. Caffeinated drinks such as coffee and soda should be avoided after noon. Alcohol can help a person fall asleep, but when the alcohol is metabolized and wears off, the patient may wake up. Sleeping pills are not a good long-term solution for sleep disturbances. Eating a large meal close to bedtime can increase your chances of developing heartburn or esophageal reflux, which can also lead to sleep difficulties.

Other medical problems can cause difficulty with sleep. Sleep apnea is a condition that causes patients to wake up because they stop breathing at night. This condition is often due to obstruction of the airway or trachea, which brings air to the lungs. The patient may have loud snoring, gasp for air, and toss and turn excessively at night. Often sleep apnea can be seen in patients who are heavier than normal. Seizures, thyroid disorders, restless leg syndrome, depression, anxiety, and many other medical conditions can interfere with sleep. If you have difficulty sleeping that persists, you may want to see a specialist in sleep medicine. This physician has special training in sleep disorders. He or she may arrange for you to sleep overnight in a sleep lab. You will be connected to special sensors that will measure your heart rate, EEG, breathing, and other parameters. You will also be videotaped to correlate your physiologic parameters with your behavior. Many patients can learn the cause of their inability to sleep by staying overnight in the sleep lab. Once a diagnosis is made, specific therapy can be prescribed to help you sleep better.

PART EIGHT

Getting Off Dialysis

Can I recover my kidney function?

What will happen if I decide to stop my dialysis treatments?

How can I get a kidney transplant?

More ...

90. Can I recover my kidney function?

This is the most frequently asked question by patients on kidney dialysis. All patients hope their kidneys will regain function and that they can stop dialysis. The chance of this happening depends on the reason your kidneys have failed. If your kidneys have failed because of acute renal failure due to a medication, an infection, uncontrolled blood pressure, or other reversible causes, recovery is a possibility. If you have acute renal failure and make a large amount of urine, say 2 quarts, you have a better chance of improving. If you are not making urine, you are less likely to recover.

Most patients with chronic progressive renal failure will not recover their renal function. This is because the process that is damaging the kidneys continues even though you began dialysis. If diabetes has affected your kidney function, the damage will continue. Patients with kidney damage tend to scar their kidneys further due to a process called **hyperfiltration**. Hyperfiltration takes place when part of a kidney is damaged by disease and is no longer able to filter blood. The remaining healthy part of the kidney filters more blood to make up for the non-functioning kidney tissue. The increase in filtration increases the pressure applied to the glomerulus, which is where the filtration takes place. This increased pressure will damage the filter, causing further kidney damage and scarring, and is harmful to the kidney. This makes the chance of renal function improving with moderate to severe kidney damage less likely. A kidney sonogram is a useful test in determining the chance of your kidneys improving. If the kidney size is small on the sonogram, this is evidence that scarring has occurred that is not reversible. Most patients with chronic renal failure will

Hyperfiltration

Occurs when a damaged kidney increases the blood flow and filtration to the remaining healthy portion of the kidney to compensate for the lost kidney function.

progress and require dialysis or a kidney transplant. Occasionally we do see a patient improving and getting off dialysis. This is a cause for celebration.

91. What will happen if I decide to stop my dialysis treatments?

It is possible to stop dialysis treatments even though renal function has not recovered. Patients stop dialysis when their medical condition deteriorates and they are suffering. Patients who stop dialysis are often elderly with many medical problems. The quality of their life has deteriorated so much that dialysis treatments and other medical treatments become intolerable. This decision is an individual one.

I had a good friend who was on hemodialysis due to kidney failure from diabetes. He also had heart problems, circulation problems, and was losing his vision. Because he lived in a rural area, he had to drive an hour to the nearest dialysis unit. This was difficult because he often felt weak after his dialysis treatments. In winter, the roads were very icy and hard to drive on. Because of his blood pressure falling during hemodialysis treatments, he switched to peritoneal dialysis at home. After a period of time, he was faced with having an amputation of his right leg due to gangrene. His vision was failing, making it more difficult to perform his peritoneal dialysis exchanges. He developed peritonitis due to *Candida*. His nephrologist wanted him to have his peritoneal catheter removed and for him to return to hemodialysis. Instead of returning to hemodialysis my friend chose to end dialysis treatments. His wife was very supportive and felt this was a good decision. Life was becoming more painful and less enjoyable. His multiple medical problems were increasing and were incurable. He stopped dialysis at age 71 and passed away peacefully at home after 10 days of stopping dialysis. This decision was a very personal one. Many patients would have continued dialysis treatments under these circumstances, even if it required spending several months in a hospital. In my many conversations with my friend over the time he was on dialysis, he emphasized quality of life as the reason to have dialysis treatments.

Stopping dialysis is usually not a painful process. The poisons and toxins from kidney failure accumulate in the system and make the patient sleepy. Patients may accumulate fluid in their legs and other parts of the body. Many patients who choose to stop their dialysis treatments feel more comfortable in a hospital or a hospice. If they have pain, breathing difficulty, or other problems, the medical staff is available to help. Patients can benefit from pain medication, oxygen, and other conservative medical therapies that will help relieve suffering.

You should discuss the issue of stopping dialysis with your nephrologist and with your family when you are doing well on dialysis. By making your thoughts and wishes known to your nephrologist and family, they will be better equipped to care for you in the future. In time, it is possible that you will become incapacitated and not fully able to make decisions on your own. Having expressed your thoughts and discussed options when you are well will help guide those you have entrusted with your well-being in the future. A **living will** is a good place to express your wishes about stopping dialysis. This legal document will

---

You should discuss the issue of stopping dialysis with your nephrologist and with your family when you are doing well on dialysis.

Living will

A legal document in which an individual states which procedures, treatments, and food he or she is willing to have in the event that he or she becomes critically ill and is unable to participate in the decision making regarding his or her medical care.

guide your family and physicians in making decisions regarding your medical care. You should identify an individual who can make decisions for you in the event that you cannot make decisions for yourself. This person is called your **healthcare proxy**. The healthcare proxy can be a spouse, blood relative, or someone not related to you. If you are unable to make your own decisions, your healthcare proxy is able to make important decisions on your behalf. It is possible that you will regain the capacity to make medical decisions. At that point, the healthcare proxy will step aside, and you will resume making decisions regarding your medical care.

Your nephrologist may decide at some point to delay your dialysis treatment because dialysis is too dangerous. If your blood pressure is too low, or if you are experiencing bleeding, a stroke, or some other emergency condition, it may be advisable to stop dialysis because the risks of dialysis outweigh the benefits. Your nephrologist will discuss this with you, your family, and your healthcare proxy to explain why it is in your best interest to delay or stop dialysis treatments. Dialysis can be reinstituted when your condition has improved.

92. How long can I live without dialysis treatments?

Living without dialysis treatments is dependent on the amount of urine you make and your residual renal function. Many patients begin dialysis when they still have some residual kidney function. They cannot live a healthy life without dialysis but can survive for a period of time. Patients who have no residual kidney function and make no urine generally can survive an average of 7

> **Healthcare proxy**
> An individual designated by a patient to make decisions regarding his or her medical care in the event that he or she is too ill to make his or her own medical decisions.

Getting Off Dialysis

to 10 days without dialysis. Every individual is different and some patients will live less time than others.

A wonderful account of stopping dialysis can be found in Art Buchwald's book *Too Soon to Say Goodbye*. Mr. Buchwald developed renal failure at 80 years of age after undergoing an angiogram for a circulation problem in his leg. After 12 hemodialysis treatments, he decided to stop dialysis against the wishes of his family. He gained some renal function and was able to survive several months and wrote a book about his experiences. His lighthearted account of dialysis, hospitals, hospices, and doctors is of value to anyone trying to decide if dialysis treatments are worthwhile. Another famous author, James Mitchner, decided to stop dialysis treatments in his 90s. As more elderly patients are treated with dialysis, the number of patients who choose to stop dialysis will increase.

Dialysis is not a very aggressive treatment. It is much less invasive than being on a ventilator, having surgery, or undergoing cardio-pulmonary resuscitation (CPR). I think of dialysis in the same category as antibiotics, intravenous fluids, blood transfusions, and food. Many family members of patients on dialysis feel they are killing their loved one if they stop dialysis treatments. This is not true. If the patient were doing well, stopping dialysis would not be an issue. The underlying disease process such as cancer, heart disease, or stroke is what is killing the patient.

Stopping dialysis is appropriate when there is no benefit to the patient and when the patient is truly suffering during treatment. Some religions and cultures do not accept the withdrawal of medical treatment. Some physicians fear that stopping dialysis in a patient who has no hope may make them more likely to face legal action. These cultural factors can make stopping dialysis more difficult. The preservation of life without regard to the quality of that life, the dignity of the patient, and the amount of suffering the person must endure is becoming more common in the United States. This problem is best addressed through education of patients and their families by the dialysis team when the patient is doing well on dialysis. A member of the clergy, sometimes called the hospital chaplain, is often available in hospitals and hospices to discuss end-of-life care with patients and their families. These clergy members have special training and can be very helpful.

93. How can I get a kidney transplant?

A successful kidney transplant is the best option for many patients with kidney failure. The transplanted kidney, like your own kidneys, works 7 days a week removing toxins and poisons from your system. It is able to make hormones such as erythropoietin, to metabolize medications, and to perform a whole host of functions we take for granted.

There are two types of kidney transplants. One is a **cadaveric kidney transplant** from a donor who has died. Each cadaveric donor can donate a kidney to two people. The donor often donates other organs such as the heart, liver, and corneas. The other type of transplant is the **living donor transplant**. This is the older type of transplant and was first performed between identical twins at the Peter Bent Brigham Hospital in Boston in 1954. The living donor donates one of his/her two kidneys to a single transplant recipient.

Cadaveric kidney transplant

A kidney transplant in which the transplanted kidney comes from a donor that has died.

Living donor transplant

A transplant in which a living person donates an organ or part of an organ. Living donor kidney transplants, partial liver transplants, and bone marrow transplants are currently being performed.

Getting Off Dialysis

Both types of transplants are very successful. The waiting list for cadaveric kidney transplants can be several years because the number of patients who want a transplant is increasing and not enough families consider organ donation when a loved one dies.

It is possible to receive a kidney transplant and never be treated with dialysis. This is the exception rather than the rule. Most patients with kidney failure will spend some time on dialysis before their kidney transplant. Arranging for a kidney transplant takes time. If the donor is a living person, they need to have a complete medical evaluation to determine if they are healthy enough to withstand surgery. They must also be free of kidney disease, infection, and cancer. The kidney is often obtained from the donor using laparoscopic surgery. Several small incisions are made in the abdomen of the patient, and the kidney can be removed through one of these small incisions. This surgery minimizes the recuperation time for the donor. The transplant recipient will also undergo an extensive evaluation by the transplant team. The kidney recipient also must be free of infection and cancer because they will receive medications to prevent the new kidney from being rejected by their body.

Rejection is a process where cells in our immune system recognize the transplanted kidney as a foreign organ. These cells will migrate to and attack the kidney. Other cells produce antibodies, which are proteins that can attach themselves to the cells of the transplanted kidney. These antibodies can injure the transplanted kidney and also make it easier for the cells of the immune system to find and destroy the new kidney. **Anti-rejection medication** must be taken by the kidney transplant recipient every day for as long as the

Rejection

An immunologic process in which the kidney transplant recipient's immune system attacks the transplant with antibodies and cells. Kidney transplant rejection impairs the ability of the transplanted kidney to remove poisons and toxins from the blood. Rejection can be diagnosed after a kidney transplant biopsy.

Anti-rejection medication

Medication used to treat acute rejection of a transplanted organ by the transplant recipient's immune system. The most common anti-rejection medications are steroids.

kidney transplant is working. The medication can make the transplant recipient more susceptible to infections such as pneumonia. They can also allow abnormal cells to grow more quickly in our bodies. If a patient has a small cancer that has not been detected, this small cancer can grow more rapidly because the anti-rejection medication inhibits the immune system's defense against these abnormal cancer cells. Anti-rejection medication can make it harder to control your blood pressure.

When you have undergone all of your tests and have satisfied the transplant center that you are healthy enough to receive a kidney transplant, you will be placed on the transplant list. Several tubes of blood will be collected from you every month to be sent to the transplant unit. These samples will enable the transplant unit to test your blood and compare it to the transplant kidney to see if you are a good match for a kidney that becomes available. The kidney must be compatible with your blood type. The transplant unit will also check to see if you are compatible with the new kidney by testing to see how similar you are genetically to the transplant kidney. The transplant unit will obtain blood tests from you and the kidney donor to measure your histocompatability antigens and can predict the chance of you rejecting your new kidney. The closer you match your new kidney at these loci, the less your chances will be of rejecting the kidney transplant.

The kidney transplant list is based on a seniority system. Available kidneys from cadaveric donors are given to the patients who have been on the transplant list the longest. An exception to this is patients who have a very close match with the kidney that is being transplanted. A patient who matches all the histo-compatability antigens of a kidney will jump the line and receive the kidney because a very well-matched kidney will have much less chance of undergoing rejection, increasing the chance that the kidney will work for a long time.

Despite the side effects of medication, the need to have surgery, and the risks of kidney rejection, kidney transplantation has become the treatment of choice in treating end-stage kidney failure. The kidney transplant recipient can live a life free from the need to have dialysis treatments. He or she can have a more varied diet. The transplant recipient is able to travel more easily without having to make special arrangements to have hemodialysis at a dialysis center or have supplies shipped to perform peritoneal dialysis. When I talk to patients who have experienced both dialysis and a kidney transplant, they all prefer the transplant as the best treatment for their kidney failure.

Erick Lucero writes:

I am hoping to get a kidney transplant. I have been on the transplant list for a year. In 2 weeks I will be going to the transplant clinic for my yearly evaluation. I hope my body accepts a new kidney. I want to live long enough to see my daughter grow up. I want to take care of my wife and daughter. My brother volunteered to donate a kidney for me. He was evaluated, but it was discovered that he had high blood sugar. The transplant team was worried that he might develop kidney problems later in life. My sister was also evaluated but was told to lose 20 pounds and come back. Several friends offered to donate a kidney, but I feel funny accepting their kidney. I do not want anyone to be hurt by donating a kidney to me.

My uncle decided that we should advertise for a kidney donor in Mexico and have the transplant there. I am worried about how safe it is to use a donor who is paid for their kidney. I am doing well on dialysis and am waiting my turn on the transplant list. The reason I want a kidney transplant is to be able to travel. I want to take my wife and daughter to Mexico on vacation. It's hard to travel when you are on hemodialysis. You have to make arrangements for your treatments in advance. If you travel outside of the United States, you have to pay for the treatments. Most insurance companies will not cover dialysis in foreign countries. They will pay for dialysis when you travel in the United States.

94. Is a kidney transplant a dangerous procedure?

Your kidney transplant will require a surgical procedure that is done under general anesthesia. This means you will not be awake during the surgery. All surgery has some risk associated with it. Before you undergo your surgery, you will have a cardiac evaluation. The biggest risk of surgery is a heart attack during or just after the surgery. Some patients with heart disease have had to have cardiac bypass surgery or cardiac stents placed to make sure their kidney transplant could be performed safely. One of the risks of transplantation is that hardening of the arteries develops more rapidly. This may be due to the anti-rejection medication that kidney transplant patients take. It is very important for patients who are considering a kidney transplant to decease their risk factors for coronary artery disease. This means stopping smoking and controlling blood pressure, cholesterol, and blood sugar if you are a diabetic. Overweight patients have an increased risk of

The over-whelming majority of patients who receive kidney transplants do well without serious complications.

heart disease. Overweight patients also have a higher risk of blood clots in their legs during and after surgery. Being able to have a kidney transplant is a good motivation for losing weight if you are heavy. Other less common complications of transplant surgery are bleeding and infection. The overwhelming majority of patients who receive kidney transplants do well without serious complications.

95. Is a kidney transplant expensive?

The average cost of a kidney transplant and the first year of medical care after the transplant is about $90,000. After the first year, the average cost of care is approximately $16,000, most of which is spent on anti-rejection medications. The cost of the surgery for the transplant is paid for by the transplant recipient's insurance. If the kidney transplant is coming from a living, related donor, the cost of the surgery for the donor is also paid for by the transplant recipient's insurance. A living-related transplant is less expensive because the kidney is more likely to function immediately after surgery and the recipient is less likely to require further dialysis. The living-related transplant recipient is more likely to have a shorter hospital stay. The cost of dialysis is about $30,000 to $50,000 a year. The break even point for a kidney transplant is 2.7 years. These numbers do not take into account the possibility that the transplant recipient may be able to return to work.

Some patients experience difficulty paying for their anti-rejection medication, which may not be covered by their insurance. Some insurance plans have maximum amounts they will pay for medications each year.

This potential problem should be discussed with the transplant team's social worker to determine if paying for medication will be a problem after the transplant. The pharmaceutical companies that manufacture anti-rejection medications have special programs for patients who are unable to afford their medications.

96. Will I reject my new kidney?

There are several types of rejections that occur after organ transplantation. **Acute rejection** is most likely to occur in the months after a kidney transplant. Rejection can be suspected when the serum creatinine, a blood test, rises. Some patients require a transplant kidney biopsy to diagnose rejection. This can be done as an outpatient procedure in many cases. Most rejection episodes respond to medications called steroids, which can be given intravenously or by mouth.

Acute rejection

Occurs when a transplant recipient's immune system attacks a transplant with antibodies and cells. It can be treated with steroids and other medication.

A more serious type of rejection is **chronic rejection**. This type of rejection occurs slowly over many years. It is also diagnosed by kidney biopsy. Unlike acute rejection, chronic rejection cannot be reversed. The function of the kidney slowly decreases with time. Chronic rejection is the reason that kidney transplants do not last forever. The average kidney transplant lasts 15 to 20 years because of chronic rejection. When kidney transplants fail, patients face a return to dialysis treatments or will consider a second kidney transplant.

Chronic rejection

A slow process mediated by the immune system in which kidney transplants become damaged and lose function over time.

97. Can I donate a kidney to my spouse?

The first kidney transplant was done between identical twins because medications to prevent rejection did not work very well. Early living-related transplants were done between parents and children or between siblings because the donor and recipient were genetically similar, which resulted in better matching and less rejection. In the 1980s, a new medication called cyclosporine was developed. This medication revolutionized the results in kidney transplantation and made liver and heart transplants more successful. At the same time there was a large increase in the number of patients waiting for kidney transplants. As a result, transplant surgeons began performing living, nonrelated kidney transplants between spouses. These transplants were successful. With the continued improvement in anti-rejection medication, more of these transplants are being done. The newspapers have reported teachers giving a kidney to a student and other inspiring examples of nonrelated kidney donations.

Another type of nonrelated transplant involves swapping kidneys between pairs of donors and recipients. Swaps work when a potential kidney donor is not compatible with a kidney recipient. If another incompatible donor and recipient can be found, it is possible for a spouse to give a kidney to a compatible recipient whose kidney donor can then donate a kidney to the incompatible partner. These kidney transplants require a great deal of counseling and psychological evaluation before they occur. They are usually done at the same time to ensure that both donors go through with the donation.

Recently a debate in the medical transplant literature has discussed the ethics of paying donors for kidney donation. In India and China, poor kidney donors regularly receive compensation for donating a kidney to an unknown recipient. Receiving payment for kidney donation beyond payment for medical expenses is considered inappropriate in the United States and most European countries. It is felt that paying for kidney donation is taking advantage of poor individuals. Many of the ethical and moral considerations regarding transplantation are affected by cultural beliefs. Japan considers using organs from deceased patients ethically wrong. Patients in Japan have had to travel to other countries to receive their transplant.

98. Can I receive more than one kidney transplant?

In a recent survey of patients on a transplant list at the University of Pennsylvania in Philadelphia, 14% of patients on the list had had a prior kidney transplant. Many patients who have had a first kidney transplant that failed have gone on to have a successful second kidney transplant. Most patients who experience the advantages of being off dialysis with a kidney transplant want to have a second transplant when they are back on dialysis. Transplant patients just feel better. They are less depressed, are able to eat a variety of foods, and are free from being attached to a machine three or more times a week on dialysis. Some patients have received more than two kidney transplants. The chances of the third and fourth transplant being successful are less than the chances of the first and second transplant being successful.

The chances of the third and fourth transplant being successful are less than the chances of the first and second transplant being successful.

It is interesting to note that some patients have received more than one type of transplant. One-third of all heart transplant patients have developed kidney failure, often due to the immunosuppressive medication they are taking to prevent the rejection of their heart transplant. If you have already received one transplant, you are on anti-rejection medication. This makes the decision to have a second organ transplant easier since you are already exposed to the side effects of the anti-rejection medication. Other common multiple organ transplants include pancreas and kidney transplants for patients with diabetes, liver and kidney transplants, and bone marrow and kidney transplants.

Transplantation is the great hope of all patients and doctors treating kidney failure. Because of the shortage of available organs, the possibility of organ transplants between species has been proposed as the solution to this important problem. Medical science has utilized tissues from other species such as pig heart valves for many years. In the 1980s several monkey-to-human transplants were performed. This was before the modern era of anti-rejection therapy. The most successful transplant functioned for 9 months. The research on cross-species transplant must make breakthroughs before this is a realistic possibility for treating patients.

99. What will I do if my kidney transplant fails?

One of the great advantages that kidney patients have is the three excellent therapies available for the treatment of kidney failure. Patients who have received a heart transplant are in serious trouble when their heart fails from rejection or other problems. They need a second transplant to survive. Liver failure patients also have no safety net. They need a second transplant when their liver transplant fails. Kidney transplant patients have the safety of dialysis. If their kidney transplant fails, they can resume dialysis treatments that are already familiar to them. The possibility of kidney transplant rejection is very frightening, but it is not medically dangerous. Kidney transplant patients are safe because they have hemodialysis and peritoneal dialysis as a backup. They will be able to resume dialysis and live a good life if their kidney transplant fails.

In the early days of kidney transplantation, patients did not have a long life expectancy. They were treated with high doses of prednisone to prevent rejection, which resulted in many complications. Children who received transplants had stunted growth. Patients developed bone problems due to osteoporosis. They developed hardening of the arteries that resulted in heart problems. They gained weight, developed diabetes, and were susceptible to infections. The present transplant patient has many fewer complications because the dose of prednisone used is very small. Some patients are treated without any prednisone being used with their anti-rejection medications, resulting in many fewer complications. Patients with kidney transplants live longer. Unfortunately transplanted kidneys eventually fail due to chronic rejection. The most successful kidney transplants last about 15 to 20 years. This means that a significant number of patients will someday be faced with resuming dialysis treatments or will need to have a second kidney transplant. Adjusting back to dialysis is not difficult for patients. They have a certain amount of depression due to the loss of their kidney. They have to adjust to a more restrictive diet. They are able to gradually stop their anti-rejection medications. Most of them go right back on the transplant list. Many others receive living-related transplants from a family member or a significant other.

The possibility of kidney transplant rejection is very frightening, but it is not medically dangerous. Kidney transplant patients are safe because they have hemodialysis and peritoneal dialysis as a backup.

Getting Off Dialysis

100. What organizations can help me cope with kidney disease?

The National Kidney Foundation (NKF) is a voluntary health organization whose mission is to prevent kidney disease and diseases of the urinary tract. It was founded in 1950 by Mr. and Mrs. Harry DeBold, who were motivated by the kidney disease of their infant son. Over the years, the National Kidney Foundation has become a powerful force that has successfully advocated for the kidney patient. Their goals are to support research, train healthcare professionals, expand patient services and community resources, educate the public, and shape healthcare policy. You probably have seen one of their walks or runs that they have organized for kidney disease at your local park. They have a wonderful Web site with information on all sorts of topics from diet to prevention of kidney failure to healthcare policy (*www.kidney.org*). The National Kidney Foundation has educational information in Spanish. They have done a wonderful job raising money for research and treatment of kidney disorders.

The American Association of Kidney Patients (AAKP) is a patient-run organization of kidney patients and health professionals. AAKP was founded by six dialysis patients after they met at a Brooklyn Hospital in 1969. From this humble start, this organization has grown into a nationwide group of patients, families, and healthcare professionals that provides support to millions of people with kidney disease. AAKP and its many activities are patient run. AAKP publishes a magazine called *Renalife* that advertises itself as "The Voice of All Kidney Patients." *Renalife* contains articles about dialysis, transplant, diet, travel, and political information written by patients and health professionals. AAKP's 35th annual convention was held in Washington, DC in August 2008. AAKP has support groups for patients and their families. The organization gives awards every year to people who have made contributions to kidney patients. AAKP is actively involved in lobbying government officials to improve the lives of patients with kidney disease. It supports research and education with grants to groups who are making advances in the care of kidney patients. AAKP has electronic newsletters as well as Healthline, a conference call designed to provide information for kidney patients. The cost of membership for patients or family members is $25 annually. More information is available from their Web site, *www.aakp.org*.

Appendix

American Association of Kidney Patients
3505 E. Frontage Road, Suite 315
Tampa, FL 33607
Phone: 1-800-749-2257
Fax: (813)-636-8122
Email: info@aakp.org
www.aakp.org

Centers for Disease Control
1600 Clifton Road
Atlanta, GA 30333
Phone: 1-800-CDC-INFO
Email: cdcinfo@cdc.gov
www.cdc.gov

Culinary Kidney Cooks
PO Box 468
Huntington Beach, CA 92648
Phone: (714) 842-4684
Fax: (714) 842-4694
Email: Eric.Brooks@CulinaryKidneyCooks.com
www.culinarykidneycooks.com

Medicare
Centers for Medicare & Medicaid Services
7500 Security Boulevard
Baltimore, MD 21244-1850
Phone: 1-800-MEDICARE
www.medicare.gov
www.cms.hhs.gov

National Center for Complementary and Alternative Medicine (NCCAM)
NCCAM
National Institutes of Health
9000 Rockville Pike
Bethesda, MD 20892
Phone: 1-888-644-6226
Fax: 1-866-464-3616
Email: info@nccam.nih.gov
http://nccam.nih.gov

National Kidney Foundation
30 East 33rd Street
New York, NY 10016
Phone: 1-800-622-9010
Fax: (212) 689-9261
www.kidney.org

The Renal Gourmet
www.kidney-cookbook.com

The Rogosin Institute
505 East 70th Street
New York, NY 10021
Phone: (212) 746-1552
Fax: (212) 288-8370
www.rogosin.org

Society for the Advancement of Blood Management
555 East Wells Street, Suite 1100
Milwaukee, WI 53202-3823
Phone: (414) 276-9339
Fax: (414) 276-3349
Email: info@sabm.org
www.sabm.org

Glossary

Access: A device that is inserted or constructed in a patient which connects the patient to the dialysis tubing and allows dialysis to take place. In hemodialysis, an access allows blood to be drawn and can be an arterial-venous (a-v) fistula, a-v graft, or a dialysis catheter. The access for peritoneal dialysis (the peritoneal dialysis catheter) is a plastic tube that allows dialysate to be instilled into the abdomen.

Access center: A medical facility that specializes in the creation and care of access for dialysis patients. The access physician uses radiology and ultrasound equipment to evaluate and improve the blood flow in a-v fistulas, a-v grafts, and catheters for hemodialysis.

Acute rejection: Occurs when a transplant recipient's immune system attacks a transplant with antibodies and cells. It can be treated with steroids and other medication.

Air bubble detector: A part of the hemodialysis machine that senses when air has entered the tubing. When air is detected, the air bubble detector quickly turns off the machine and clamps the tubing to prevent it from going into the patient.

Albumin: A water-soluble protein found in the blood normally in very minute amounts. Patients with kidney disease often have albumin in their urine because the albumin leaks through the damaged kidneys into the urine.

Alternative medicine: A medical discipline that uses natural products and diet to treat medical illness.

American Society of Nephrology (ASN): A national organization of physicians and scientists founded in 1966 to study and treat kidney disease.

Amino acids: Organic acids that are the building blocks of proteins.

Anemia: A decrease in the number of red blood cells present in the blood, which can be due to blood loss or a decreased production of red blood cells due to iron deficiency, poor nutrition, or disease. Decreased red blood cell survival occurs in kidney disease. Symptoms of anemia include fatigue, weakness, and shortness of breath on exertion.

Angina: Chest pain due to lack of blood to the heart that is often described as a squeezing pain or heaviness. Angina can be precipitated by exercise and is relieved by rest and nitroglycerin, a medication that can be taken intravenously or orally.

Angioedema: A serious allergic reaction characterized by swelling of a body part, often the face or lips.

Angioplasty: A medical procedure in which a balloon catheter is inserted into a blood vessel or dialysis access. When the balloon is inflated, it opens a blockage in the blood vessel to improve blood flow.

Angiotensin: A polypeptide produced in the kidney, which causes blood pressure to rise.

Angiotensin-converting enzyme inhibitors (ACE inhibitors): A class of medications that is useful in treating high blood pressure, stabilizing kidney disease, and improving patients with congestive heart failure. ACE inhibitors stabilize kidney disease by decreasing the amount of protein in the urine and decreasing the damage done by elevated blood pressure.

Angiotensin receptor blocker (ARB): A class of medications that has similar properties to ACE inhibitors. ARBs can treat high blood pressure, stabilize

kidney disease, decrease protein in the urine, and treat congestive heart failure.

Anti-rejection medication: Medication used to treat acute rejection of a transplanted organ by the transplant recipient's immune system. The most common anti-rejection medications are steroids.

Arterial-venuous (a-v) fistula: A tube that connects an artery to a vein and is constructed by a vascular surgeon. When mature, the a-v fistula can have needles inserted into it to carry blood through plastic tubing to and from the hemodialysis machine.

Arterial-venuous (a-v) graft: A length of gortex tubing connected between an artery and a vein that is created by a vascular surgeon. The a-v graft is tunneled under the skin to allow needles to be inserted into it to carry blood through plastic tubing to the hemodialysis machine.

Atherosclerosis: A disease process that involves deposition of cholesterol in the walls of arteries, causing narrowing of the arteries. This can cause blood to clot, further reducing blood flow. Atherosclerosis decreases the amount of blood that can flow to the organs of the body and is increased by an elevated blood pressure, uncontrolled diabetes, smoking, and an elevated cholesterol level.

Autosomal dominant polycystic kidney disease (ADPKD): The most common form of inherited kidney disease. Patients inherit the gene from either parent and many cysts form in the kidneys.

Bacillus Calmette-Guerin (BCG): A tuberculosis vaccine given to children in many countries with a high prevalence of tuberculosis. Patients who have received BCG will often have a positive skin test for tuberculosis for the rest of their lives.

Beta blockers: A class of medication named for its ability to block beta receptors in the heart, blood vessels, and other organs. Beta blockers are used to treat chest pain or angina, congestive heart failure, high blood pressure, and migraine headaches.

Bicarbonate: A salt of carbonic acid that acts as an important buffer to help keep our blood from becoming too acidic.

Blood pump: A circular device that is easily visible on the front of every hemodialysis machine. This roller pump compresses plastic tubing that propels blood from the patient to the dialysis machine and back to the patient.

Blood urea nitrogen (BUN): A common blood test used to screen patients for kidney disease. An elevated BUN can indicate decreased kidney function.

Bright's Disease: An old term, named after Dr. Richard Bright (1789-1858) who first described the association of protein in the urine with kidney disease and renal failure. Although this term is no longer used clinically, it reminds us of Dr.

Bright's great contribution to the treatment of kidney disease.

Bruit: A French word meaning "noise" that is used to describe the sound that blood makes when rushing through a blood vessel or dialysis access. A bruit can be heard with a stethoscope or by holding the access against your ear. A bruit heard in an a-v fistula or a-v graft signifies that blood is flowing through the access and that it is working.

Cadaveric kidney transplant: A kidney transplant in which the transplanted kidney comes from a donor that has died.

Calcium: A mineral found in our bones, blood, and cells.

Calculus: Comes from the Latin word for stone. A kidney stone is sometimes referred to as a calculus. The term is also used by dentists to describe a calcified layer of saliva, bacteria, protein, and sugar covering the teeth.

Cannulation: The insertion of needles into the dialysis access to obtain blood for hemodialysis.

Catheter: A plastic tube used for dialysis. Catheters are inserted into blood vessels to obtain blood for hemodialysis treatments. Peritoneal dialysis catheters are inserted in the abdomen, and are used to instill and drain dialysate into and out of the abdomen during peritoneal dialysis treatments.

Cellcept (mycophenolate mofetil): An immunosuppressant medication that inhibits the proliferation of T and

B lymphocytes, which are important cells in the rejection of kidney transplants. Cellcept is used with other medications to prevent rejection in kidney and other organ transplants. It is also used alone in the treatment of kidney disease due to lupus erythematosus. Cellcept can be taken orally or intravenously.

Cholesterol: A substance manufactured in the liver or ingested that is present in the blood, liver, brain, and other organs. When deposited in blood vessels, cholesterol can lead to atherosclerosis.

Chronic rejection: A slow process mediated by the immune system in which kidney transplants become damaged and lose function over time.

Computerized axial tomography (CT) scan: A computer generated three-dimensional x-ray picture of part of the body used for the diagnosis of disease. It is sometimes called a CT scan.

Continuous ambulatory peritoneal dialysis (CAPD): A home dialysis procedure taught to patients who perform their own peritoneal dialysis, CAPD involves the instillation by gravity of dialysate through a catheter into the abdomen. The fluid remains in the abdomen for a time, allowing poisons and toxins to accumulate in the dialysate. The dialysate is then drained and discarded, and fresh dialysate is instilled.

Continuous cyclical peritoneal dialysis (CCPD): A home peritoneal dialysis procedure that uses a cycler to instill and drain fluid into the abdomen. The cycler can perform peritoneal dialysis while the patient is sleeping.

Creatinine: A substance released into the blood from our muscles. Since it is eliminated from the body by the kidneys, a decrease in kidney function results in an elevation of creatinine in the blood. An elevated creatinine blood test is an indication of decreased kidney function.

Cycler: A machine used to automate peritoneal dialysis by performing the exchange of peritoneal dialysis fluid.

Cyclosporine: A medication, originally isolated from fungi, that is used in preventing the rejection of kidney and other organ transplants. Cyclosporine can also be used to treat some kidney diseases.

Cystoscopy: A surgical procedure performed by a urologist in which a small fiber-optic tube called a cystoscope is inserted through the urethra into the bladder. The urologist can diagnose tumors of the bladder and can perform biopsies and other procedures through the cystoscope.

Depression: A medical term used to describe feelings of intense sadness, loss of interest in activities of daily life, and a decreased appetite and sense of well-being.

Dextrose: A sugar added to peritoneal dialysis solutions to help remove fluid from the body. It is also added to intravenous fluids to provide calories for nutrition.

Diabetes: A disease characterized by an elevation of the glucose level in the blood. This can be caused by a decrease in insulin production by the pancreas or a defect in the insulin receptor.

Diabetes nurse educator: A nurse who has obtained special training and certification in the evaluation and education of patients with diabetes.

Dialysate: A fluid containing sodium, calcium, bicarbonate, and other substances that is used to remove toxins and poisons during dialysis. Different dialysate solutions are used in hemodialysis and peritoneal dialysis.

Dialysis: A scientific term for the movement of substances across a membrane by a process called diffusion.

Dialysis partner: A person who has received special training in performing hemodialysis or peritoneal dialysis and who assists you in performing dialysis at home.

Dialysis technician: A healthcare worker who works in the hemodialysis unit under the supervision of a registered nurse. Dialysis technicians can institute hemodialysis by inserting needles into the access, and can also monitor the dialysis treatment, measure blood pressure, and help educate dialysis patients regarding their treatment, but they are not allowed to administer medication.

Dialyzer: A medical device that contains the dialysis membrane. It is connected to tubing that allows blood to flow into the dialyzer on one side of the membrane and then back to the patient. Dialysate flows on the other side of the membrane, and poisons and toxins move from the blood across the membrane into the dialysate, which is then discarded.

Dietitian: A registered health professional who has special training in nutrition. Dietitians advise patients on which foods to eat and which to avoid based upon their individual needs. They use monthly laboratory tests to monitor the patient's progress.

Disequilibrium syndrome: A syndrome in which the rapid removal of poisons and toxins during hemodialysis results in less toxins being present in the blood than in the brain. This difference causes water to leave the blood stream and enter the central nervous system, leading to brain swelling. Symptoms include headache, nausea, vomiting, fatigue, and weakness. Most of these symptoms are gone by the next day. A severe disequilibrium syndrome can cause seizures and coma.

Dry weight: The body weight of hemodialysis patients at the end of their hemodialysis treatment. The dry weight is determined by removing fluid until the blood pressure begins to fall.

Edema: The medical term for fluid that collects in an area of the body. The most common location for edema is in the legs. The legs appear swollen, especially after walking around. The edema decreases after a night's sleep because it has moved to other areas of the body. Other areas that can collect fluid are the lungs and abdomen.

Electrocardiogram (EKG): A medical test in which electrical impulses generated by the heart are recorded by attaching electrodes to the arms, legs, and chest.

Electroencephalogram (EEG): A medical test in which electrical impulses generated by the brain are recorded by attaching electrodes to the scalp.

Endocrinologist: A physician who has trained in internal medicine and who has received additional training in the treatment of patients with diabetes, thyroid disease, parathyroid disease, and other glandular disorders.

Eosinophils: White blood cells produced by the bone marrow that are normally found in the blood. During allergic reactions, the number of eosinophils increases.

Erythropoietin: A hormone produced by the kidneys that signals the bone marrow to produce more red blood cells. In kidney disease, less erythropoietin is produced and anemia can occur. Erythropoietin can be given by injection to treat anemia.

Exchange: A term used in peritoneal dialysis that describes fluid being drained using plastic tubing from the abdomen into a collection bag. New peritoneal dialysate is infused by gravity into the abdomen.

Exit site care: Exit site care involves swabbing the area where the peritoneal dialysis catheter exits the skin with an antiseptic solution and covering the exit site with a clean sterile dressing.

Focal segmental glomerular sclerosis (FSGS): The most common primary kidney disease in black and Hispanic patients in the United States; it is also found in patients from other ethnic backgrounds. FSGS is suspected when protein is found in the urine and is diagnosed after performing a kidney biopsy.

Gastroenterologist: A physician who has received training in internal medicine and who has had additional training in the diagnosis and treatment of disorders of the digestive system.

Glomerulonephritis: An inflammation of the filter or glomerulus of the kidney caused by many diseases.

Glomerulus: The part of the kidney composed of small blood vessels that filters the blood to produce urine.

Glycogen: A polysaccharide composed of glucose, which is the principal storage unit of carbohydrates in the body.

Health maintenance organization (HMO): An organization that manages a patient's health care for a health insurance company. A patient who is a member of an HMO can select a doctor from a panel available. If they go to a doctor outside of the panel, they may have to pay to see that physician and their health insurance may not reimburse them. The HMO may require approval before your doctor can order certain tests or medications and may have agreements with dialysis units, limiting your choice in where you can receive your dialysis treatments or kidney transplant. By managing health care, the HMO can obtain affordable health care for its patients.

Healthcare proxy: An individual designated by a patient to make decisions regarding his or her medical care in the event that he or she is too ill to make his or her own medical decisions.

Hemodialysis: A medical treatment in which blood is removed from the patient with needles and plastic tubing and pumped past the dialysis membrane. Poisons and toxins cross the dialysis membrane into the dialysate, which is then discarded, and the blood is returned to the patient. A typical hemodialysis treatment lasts four hours.

Heparin: An acid that occurs naturally in the liver and lungs that can be purified and used as a medication to prevent blood from clotting. Heparin is used in hemodialysis to prevent blood from clotting in the plastic tubing and when exposed to the dialysis membrane. It can also be injected into the peritoneal dialysis fluid to prevent clots from blocking the peritoneal dialysis catheter.

Hepatitis B vaccine: A vaccine given to patients in a series of three intramuscular injections. The vaccine stimulates the body to produce antibodies against Hepatitis B. It is recommended for children as part of their routine vaccinations. Patients with kidney disease who have not received the Hepatitis B vaccine should be vaccinated.

High-biologic-value protein: Proteins found in foods such as eggs, fish, poultry, soy products, and meat. High-biologic-value proteins are easily digestible and are rich in the ten essential amino acids that our body cannot make.

High-density lipoprotein (HDL): The "good cholesterol" in our blood that protects us from heart disease and other vascular problems. A high level of HDL is protective, and it can be increased by exercising, eating foods such as garlic and onions, and by taking certain medications.

High flux dialysis: A procedure that uses high blood flows and large dialysis membranes to remove poisons and toxins in a shorter dialysis treatment, although short dialysis treatments are no longer recommended. The experience with high flux dialysis helped kidney doctors improve dialysis treatments by removing more toxins during regular hemodialysis treatments.

Home dialysis: Includes hemodialysis treatments performed by the patient with the help of another person in the family, and also peritoneal dialysis. Occasionally, patients have insurance that covers a hemodialysis nurse or technician to perform their hemodialysis at home.

Horseshoe kidney: A medical condition in which the right and left kidneys are fused at the upper or lower pole. Ninety percent of horseshoe kidneys are fused at the lower pole. The horseshoe kidney is capable of normal kidney function and is usually found when a CT scan or ultrasound (sonogram) is performed for abdominal pain or other symptoms. Patients with a horseshoe kidney are not predisposed to kidney disease.

Human immunodeficiency virus (HIV): The etiologic virus in HIV/AIDS infection. HIV can be transmitted through blood transfusion, intravenous drug use, sexual activity, and through a needle stick. HIV cannot be transmitted during dialysis treatments.

Hyperfiltration: Occurs when a damaged kidney increases the blood flow and filtration to the remaining healthy portion of the kidney to compensate for the lost kidney function.

Hyperparathyroidism: A condition in which the four parathyroid glands, located next to the thyroid gland in the neck, increase their production of the parathyroid hormone (PTH). This is due to a low blood calcium level that is caused by elevated phosphorus production and low Vitamin D production. Hyperparathyroidism is treated by lowering phosphorus levels with dietary modifications and phosphate binders, and by taking medication to suppress the production of parathyroid hormone. Occasionally, patients have three-and-a-half of their parathyroid glands removed by surgery.

Hypertension: A condition in which the blood pressure is elevated on two or more occasions. High blood pressure can be caused by kidney disease and is associated with increased body weight. Treatment of hypertension includes diet and lifestyle modification and medication.

Hypertrophy: An increase in the size of the kidney.

Ideal body weight: Ideal body weight is dependent upon your age, height, body, build, and sex, and is based on the measured average weight of normal individuals. Ideal body weights can be found in published tables, which are available from your kidney dietitian.

IgA nephropathy: A disease of the kidney that often presents with blood and protein in the urine. The immunoglobulin IgA is seen in the kidney on biopsy.

Immunosuppressive therapy: Immunosuppressive therapy works by suppressing the activity of the cells and antibodies of the immune system. In the treatment of some kidney diseases, immunosuppressive medicines are given intravenously or orally to decrease the immune response. Kidney transplant patients also need immunosuppressive medications to prevent rejection of the transplant.

Insensible fluid loss: The fluid that leaves the body in the form of water vapor from the lungs, sweat, and fluid in stool. The amount of insensible fluid loss is about 2 to 3 cups every day.

Internist: A doctor who has had specialized training in internal medicine. The internist is trained in the prevention, diagnosis, and treatment of disease in adults. An internist can determine if you have kidney disease, begin treatment, and refer you to an appropriate kidney doctor.

Ischemia: A decrease or lack of blood flow to an organ in the body causing damage or organ dysfunction.

Kayexalate (sodium polystyrene): A medication that is taken orally and is used to treat an elevated potassium level. Kayexalate comes as a powder which can be mixed in water or juice and is often given with a sugar called sorbitol to cause diarrhea to eliminate the kayexalate that binds potassium in stool.

Kidney biopsy: A test that can diagnose the cause of kidney failure. It is an outpatient procedure performed by an invasive radiologist or nephrologist in which the exact location of one of your kidneys is visualized with a sonogram or CT scan. Local anesthesia is administered with lidocaine and a small needle is inserted into one kidney. A small piece of kidney tissue is then removed and examined under the microscope by a renal pathologist who will report the diagnosis to your nephrologist.

Kidney cyst: A fluid-filled structure commonly discovered by renal ultrasound (sonogram) or CT scan. Renal cysts are common as we age and are usually benign. Patients with polycystic kidney disease have many cysts that will eventually damage the kidneys and lead to kidney failure.

Kidney stone: Seventy five percent of kidney stones are made up of calcium. They form when there is too much calcium in the urine. Other kidney stones are made of uric acid, cystine, or other substances. Kidney stones may be diagnosed after patients experience severe pain and are often found on kidney sonograms or CT scans.

Kidney transplant rejection: Occurs when the transplant recipient's immune system attacks the new kidney with antibodies and cells; it can be reversed with anti-rejection medication. Chronic rejection occurs over time and is difficult to treat. Kidney transplant rejection can be diagnosed after a biopsy of the transplanted kidney.

Kidney tubule: Tubes composed of cells that carry urine filtered by the glomerulus to the collecting system. Renal tubular cells secrete potassium and acids and re-absorb sodium, bicarbonate, and other substances.

Kidneys: Two fist-sized organs located in the posterior upper abdomen that maintain fluid and salt balance and detoxify the blood by eliminating toxins and poisons from the body in the urine.

Laparoscopic surgery: Surgery performed under general anesthesia by inserting fiber-optic tubes through several small incisions.

Licensed practical nurse (LPN): A healthcare professional who has completed a nursing program and passed a licensing exam. An LPN works under the supervision of registered nurses and physicians.

Lipid profile (lipid panel): A lipid profile is a series of blood tests that include total cholesterol, HDL cholesterol, LDL cholesterol, and triglycerides. It is used to evaluate patients for their risk of developing atherosclerosis.

Living donor transplant: A transplant in which a living person donates an organ or part of an organ. Living donor kidney transplants, partial liver transplants, and bone marrow transplants are currently being performed.

Living will: A legal document in which an individual states which procedures, treatments, and food he or she is willing to have in the event that he or she becomes critically ill and is unable to participate in the decision making regarding his or her medical care.

Low-density lipoproteins (LDL): Composed of proteins, triglycerides, and cholesterol bound together in the blood. A high LDL level is associated with atherosclerosis.

Lupus erythematosus: A disease in which the body's immune system attacks its own organs. Also called systemic lupus erythematosus (SLE).

Medicaid: A federally-funded insurance program that is administered by the states to provide medical services, medications, and transportation to medical treatments for patients who have limited monetary resources.

Medicare: A federally-funded program that provides medical treatments and services to patients over the age of 65 and to patients who are younger than 65 and disabled.

Meninges: The three membranes that cover the brain and spinal cord. The meninges form a barrier between the central nervous system and the rest of the body, known as the blood-brain barrier.

Metabolic bone disease: Bone disease in renal patients is caused by reabsorption of bone by cells called osteoclasts whose growth is stimulated by PTH. Patients with bone disease can have bone pain and are more prone to fractures. Also called renal osteodystrophy.

Microalbumin: A test designed to detect very small elevated amounts of the protein albumin in the urine that are not able to be detected by a routine urine analysis.

Muscle wasting: A decrease in the size of the muscles of the body due to poor nutrition or medical illness.

Nephrologist: A physician who has completed four years of medical school, three years of training in internal medicine, and two or more additional years of specialized training in the diagnosis and management of diseases of the kidney.

Nephrology fellow: A doctor who has completed training in internal medicine and is receiving additional training in the evaluation and treatment of kidney diseases, dialysis, and kidney transplantation.

Nephron: The functional unit of the kidney. Our kidneys contain about two million nephrons, which each consist of a glomerulus that filters the blood, kidney tubules that secrete and absorb substances, and a collecting system to transport urine to the renal pelvis.

Neuropathy: Damage to the peripheral nerves of the body. Symptoms include tingling in the hands and feet, weakness, and numbness.

Nocturnal hemodialysis: Hemodialysis treatments done at night six or seven days a week at the patient's home while the patient is asleep. Nocturnal hemodialysis treatments utilize a lower blood pump flow and a longer duration of treatment time to achieve gentle treatments with better clearance of toxins and poisons.

Nurse practitioner: A nurse who has received additional training in the diagnosis and treatment of diseases. The nurse practitioner is able to prescribe medication and perform medical procedures.

Omega 3 fatty acids: A family of unsaturated fatty acids that is thought to decrease the risk of ather-

osclerosis. They have also been used to treat IgA nephropathy, which can cause kidney failure.

Parathyroid hormone (PTH): A hormone made and released by the chief cells of the four parathyroid glands found in the neck to regulate calcium metabolism.

Peripheral nervous system: Nerves that leave the spinal cord and go to the organs, muscles, and skin. These nerves carry information from the brain to the body, and also bring information back to the brain.

Peritoneal dialysis: Dialysis treatments that use the patient's peritoneal membrane in the abdomen as a dialysis membrane to remove toxins and wastes from the body.

Peritonitis: An inflammation of the peritoneal membrane, which covers the intestines, caused by infection.

Phosphate binder: Medications taken by mouth at mealtimes to decrease the absorption of phosphorus contained in food.

Physician's assistant: A member of the healthcare team who works under the supervision of a physician and diagnoses and manages medical problems.

Podiatrist: A healthcare professional who is trained in the diagnosis and treatment of disorders of the feet.

Psychologist: A healthcare professional who works with patients on their mental health problems including depression and anxiety.

Recirculation: Occurs during hemodialysis treatments when blood that has gone through the dialysis machine does not mix with the patient's blood but returns to the dialysis machine.

Red blood cells: Cells made by the bone marrow that contain an oxygen transport protein called hemoglobin, which causes blood to appear red. Red blood cells carry oxygen from the lungs to other organs through the circulatory system.

Registered nurse (RN): A healthcare professional who has graduated from a nursing program and passed state qualifying examinations.

Rejection: An immunologic process in which the kidney transplant recipient's immune system attacks the transplant with antibodies and cells. Kidney transplant rejection impairs the ability of the transplanted kidney to remove poisons and toxins from the blood. Rejection can be diagnosed after a kidney transplant biopsy.

Renal diet: A diet that avoids foods that contain sodium, potassium, and phosphorus, and limits the amount of fluid intake.

Renal replacement therapy: Renal replacement therapy replaces kidney function by removing toxins, poisons, salts, fluid, and medications from the body. Renal replacement therapies for patients outside of the hospital include hemodialysis, peritoneal dialysis, and kidney transplant. Patients in intensive care units in hospital can also receive continuous renal replacement therapies such as continuous venovenous hemofiltration (CVVH).

Reverse osmosis (RO): A water purification technique in which water is pushed through a membrane at high pressure to remove impurities. Water treated with reverse osmosis is then used to make dialysate for hemodialysis.

Semipermeable membrane: A membrane used for dialysis that allows small substances such as salts, phosphorus, glucose, and water to pass through while blocking larger substances and cells.

Serum albumin: A protein that constitutes more than one half of the protein found in the blood. During kidney disease, albumin can be lost in the urine resulting in a decreased serum albumin level. The serum albumin is also low in liver disease and malnutrition.

Serum creatinine: A blood test used to screen patients for kidney disease. Creatinine is a breakdown product of muscle. When the kidney function is decreased, the kidneys filter less creatinine and the serum creatinine level rises.

Shunt: An old term used to describe an access used to obtain blood for hemodialysis. It initially referred to the Quinton-Scribner shunt first used in the 1960s. Today, the term includes the a-v fistula and a-v graft which "shunt" blood from the artery to the vein, bypassing the small capillaries.

Sickle cell anemia: An inherited anemia that results in red blood cells forming a crescent shape. Sickle cells block small vessels and can result in injury to the bones, heart, lungs, and kidneys.

Social worker: A licensed professional who is part of the multidisciplinary team at the dialysis unit. The social worker assists patients with emotional, financial, and social issues, and also provides education and referrals to community resources. A nephrology social worker specializes in services that support patients and families who are adjusting to the major lifestyle changes that are caused by end stage renal disease.

Sonogram: A medical test in which sound waves are used to obtain pictures of organs in the body. A kidney sonogram requires no injections of substances or exposure to radiation. Also known as an ultrasound.

Steal syndrome: A syndrome that occurs when too much blood is taken away from the arm or hand by an a-v fistula or a-v graft. The blood goes from the artery to the vein, bypassing the capillaries to the hand or arm, resulting in coolness, pain, and sometimes loss of function of the hand.

Stent: A medical device that looks like a hollow tube. Stents are inserted across blocked blood arteries to the heart, kidneys, and other organs to increase the blood flow. Other kinds of stents are also used to treat blockages in the ureters that transport urine from the kidneys to the bladder.

Thrill: A vibration felt over an a-v fistula or a-v graft caused by blood flowing through the a-v access. A thrill is a sign that the access is working.

Thrombectomy: A procedure in which a blood clot that is blocking a blood vessel or an a-v access is removed or dissolved with medication. It allows blood to flow through the hemodialysis access so it can be used for hemodialysis.

Tolerance: The need for an increasing amount of medication to produce the same effect over time. A common example is the need to use more pain medication to relieve chronic pain.

Transplant list: A list of patients who have successfully completed their transplant evaluation and who are waiting for a cadaveric kidney transplant.

Twenty-four hour urine collection: A test used to measure the amount of protein that a patient is losing in the urine and which also measures the renal function of the patient. The patient typically voids, and then collects all of his or her urine from 8 AM to 8 AM the following day.

Ultrasound: An ultrasound, also known as a sonogram, is a diagnostic test that bounces sound waves off internal organs, such as the kidneys, to obtain a picture of them. Ultrasound does not require x-rays, injection, or dye, and is safe for pregnant patients.

Universal precautions: Wearing medical gloves, goggles, and face shields to avoid contact with body fluids such as blood and peritoneal fluid. Universal precautions protect us from the risk of transmission of blood-borne diseases such as hepatitis and HIV-AIDS.

Urea reduction ratio (URR): A mathematical calculation using the BUN done before and after dialysis that is used to measure the amount of hemodialysis a patient is receiving.

Uremia: Symptoms caused by kidney failure that include loss of appetite, itching, hiccups, nausea, vomiting, seizures, and lethargy.

Uremic neuropathy: Damage to nerves that is caused by the toxins and poisons that build up in the blood in kidney failure. Typical symptoms of uremic neuropathy are tingling or numbness in the feet and hands. Uremic neuropathy is treated by increasing the amount of dialysis that the patient is receiving to remove the build-up of toxins and poisons. Medications are sometimes used to treat the symptoms of uremic neuropathy.

Ureter: A tube that caries urine from the kidney to the bladder.

Urethra: A tube that carries urine from the bladder to the outside of the patient.

Urine analysis: A common screening test that looks for the presence of protein, glucose, and cells in the urine. It can help determine if further tests for kidney disease are indicated.

Urologist: A physician who specializes in the diagnosis and treatment of diseases of the kidney and urinary tract. Urologists have training in surgical procedures used in the treatment of prostate problems, tumors of the urinary tract, and the removal of kidney stones.

Index

Index